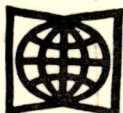

THE BIRTH OF A FATHER

New Fathers Talk About Pregnancy, Childbirth, and the First Three Months

by Cecilia Worth

A Sun Words Book

McGraw-Hill Book Company

New York	St. Louis	San Francisco	Auckland	Bogotá	Hamburg
London	Madrid	Mexico	Milan	Montreal	New Delhi	Panama
Paris	São Paulo	Singapore	Sydney	Tokyo	Toronto

1 2 3 4 5 6 7 8 9 F G R F G R 8 9 0 9 8

ISBN 0-07-071826-1{H.C.}

ISBN 0-07-071825-3{PBK.}

LIBRARY OF CONGRESS CATALOGING-IN-PUBLICATION DATA

Worth, Cecilia.
    The birth of a father.
    (A Sun words book)
    1. Pregnancy.   2. Childbirth.   3. Infants—Care.
4. Fathers—Attitudes.   5. Fathers—Interviews.
I. Title.
RG525.W68   1988   306.8'742   87-3088
ISBN 0-07-071826-1
ISBN 0-07-071825-3 (pbk.)

Edited by Sandra Oddo

Design by Richards Steinbock

Dedicated with love to my father,
who, being the person that he is,
gave me many of the values
that brought me today's successes.

Written with respect, gratitude and affection
for these men who moved and inspired me
with their curiosity concerning the unknown,
their willingness to take risks,
and their courage to be themselves.

Contents

Introduction:
The Birth of a Book

A man, sandy-haired and grinning broadly under his jaunty red cap, strode forward from behind the supermarket meat counter and shook my hand enthusiastically.

"Remember me?" he asked. "I'm one of your fathers!"

"Of course," I exclaimed, delighted. "What a pleasure to see you! Your daughter must be three years old now."

Over the years, unexpected meetings and impromptu conversations with men who had partnered their pregnant wives through my classes in prepared childbirth have been a special experience.

Glowing, this thirty-year-old father announced that by now he had a second child. Then, taking a deep breath, he became serious.

"You know," he said earnestly, "I still can't believe what I went through with that first baby. I couldn't express it then, but that year was the shock of my life. I'd come home from work at night, the house a mess, the baby screaming, my wife exhausted, in tears, still wearing her nightgown. I'd take over—put the baby to bed, wash the dishes, try to get my wife to relax—but all the time I'd be thinking I'd lost her, that having a baby had been a terrible mistake."

Oblivious to the shoppers strolling by, he leaned against the counter, wearing his loose butcher's coat, and talked on and on about the flood of doubts and fears, surprises, and worries during the year when he became a father. "I never told her how I felt, even to this day. The man is supposed to be the strong one, right? But some evenings I had to get out of there. I'd pretend I needed cigarettes and take off in my truck so I could be alone and think. Once I pulled off the road, put my head down on the steering wheel and cried."

Similar confessions from other first-time fathers have been shared with me many, many times in my twenty years of teaching courses for expectant and new parents. When their wives became pregnant, these men had no advance notice that they would find themselves riding emotional roller coasters—worrying, uncertain, peevish, resentful, jealous, scared, sad, vulnerable, moved to unfamiliar tears and tenderness—intense responses that profoundly influenced their self-images.

During pregnancy and the arrival of a new baby, women, not men, traditionally bask in the spotlight of attention. Men, seen in a supporting role at best, are shunted to the sidelines. Worse, they often are reduced to cliché status by cartoons, movies, television, and novels that portray them as excited bumblers, dashing nervously to the all-night deli for ice cream and pickles, fumbling awkwardly through diaper changes.

Guided only by such superficial characterizations, rarely viewed as people reacting to a major life change, expectant and new fathers have no way to cope with the powerful barrage of emotions that is as normal for them as it is for their mates, despite the old-fashioned notion that males are less emotionally vulnerable than females.

Men are trained from childhood to be calm, clear, and composed—rocks of Gibraltar—or at least to appear to be. To complicate matters, they are also taught to hide what they are feeling. So, supposing what they go through to be unique, thinking other fathers are really as assured as they seem, many of the men I met kept the emotionally troubling aspects of becoming a father to themselves, privately agonizing "What's the matter with me?" As a result, they often avoided reaching for the support they might otherwise have received from one another, from wives, families, friends, even from the medical people involved in mothers' care.

The secrecy works in reverse, too. Few of these people, focused as they are on the mother, think to volunteer support, unaware that it is needed. That any father winds up enduring this emotional time in solitude is more than unfortunate. It is tragic.

The men who have talked with me about this crucial period in their lives were from all walks of life. Barriers of background, education, and class evaporated before their universal experience. "How do other guys handle this?" they wanted to know. As I listened, I used to think, "If only other men could hear what these men are saying."

And so the idea for a book was born, a book that would come straight from the fathers themselves, quoting them, giving readers the sense of having dropped in on lively, enlightening, honest discussions among men reviewing the year they became fathers.

Here it is. It contains a sampling of the words and experiences of thousands of men who attended my classes and who spoke with me or mailed me accounts afterward. As you read, you will meet a small group of men whose stories are typical of those told to me by so many fathers.

I was always deeply touched to be entrusted with this most personal information. At group interviews, which came about as a result of questionnaires developed specifically for this book, men who started out as strangers to one another quickly lost their self-consciousness and talked as if the conversation were a relay race, words tumbling out.

An important key to this free flow of sharing was the purpose of the meetings. We were doing this to put together information that would enlighten and encourage other expectant and new fathers whom we would probably never meet, but to whom we related empathetically. We wanted to assure them that they were not alone. United by such a philanthropic focus, the men at the meetings felt, not like specimens under a microscope, but like comrades.

There were further dividends. The bull sessions were a catharsis that emphasized the normalcy of these fathers' experiences. In addition the men discovered that, by talking together and reflecting on one another's experiences and points of view, they uncovered parts of themselves they hadn't known existed. Seeing the process of becoming fathers more completely, they came to understand and appreciate themselves more fully.

The fathers represented in this book are in committed relationships, some married, some not. They are men who wanted children, or at least came to a clear decision to have them after giving serious thought to starting a family. The pregnancies were free from extreme problems. The book does not include single fathers, men whose children were unwanted, very young or much older fathers—that is, men whose reactions toward fatherhood are focused on the specifics of their particular situations. But even fathers in special circumstances may see themselves in much of what is expressed here. Without a doubt, all men entering fatherhood have much in common.

The book parallels the three main stages of the year a baby arrives: pregnancy, birth, and the first three months with the new infant. Each period has its own message and impact. All three are linked in a unique adventure.

As you travel this amazing journey with these men, keep in mind that what they describe is not how a father *should* feel, but how he *might* feel. Their experiences offer, not predictions, but glimpses of possibilities. Men can be reassured by these fathers, and learn as they did. They can count themselves among many normal, responsive, sensitive men—courageous pioneers who welcome the barrage of feelings triggered by pregnancy, birth, and new fatherhood as a chance to learn about themselves, to express these feelings as part of who they are, and perhaps to become better fathers.

PREGNANCY

"How would I advise other men during their pregnancies? I would say, 'Get your act together about yourself. Feel strong about who you are. Go for exactly what you want. Let people know. Be honest and clear. Then you'll be okay.' What causes difficulty is when you are hazy about what works for you."

1 Receiving the News

The pregnancy test is positive. Fatherhood is certain. In less than nine months the man hearing this news will hold his own baby in his arms. Incredible? It seems so. But true? Absolutely! A reason to celebrate? Immediately! A reason to worry? Definitely! Any questions? Only several dozen!

The response from men reminiscing about the year each became a father was universal. One after another agreed that the confirmation of pregnancy had set off a whirlwind of intense emotions, whether they had been hoping passionately for a baby or were caught by surprise.

Within their common experience, however, each man's reaction was, and is, distinctly individual.

Clarence, a tall, lanky man trained as a lighting engineer, generally quiet and reserved, smiled as he recalled his response. He felt jubilant, lifted from the ordinary to a connection with the miraculous.

> "I was ecstatic. I thought my wife was great. I thought I was great. Such pride! Immortality was mine. I had created life! I wanted to crow like a rooster at the rising sun. I walked—ran!—into town and told everyone I met. Everyone!"

For Craig, a musician whose soft speaking voice is a surprising counterpoint to his nervous, intense manner, pregnancy was a confirmation of manhood.

> "I was overjoyed and relieved at the same time. In a remote part of me I'd always questioned my fertility."

The reality of pregnancy can be difficult to comprehend. Andre, who owns and runs a bookstore, had lived happily for several years with the woman who would now bear their child. A romantic at heart, he had been enthusiastic about the idea of pregnancy, but was disappointed with the early reality.

"There was nothing to see, touch, or hear. It seemed unreal, a dream almost," he explained.

Some newly expectant fathers react with fear and uncertainty, like Scott, a red-haired, blue-eyed, shy-mannered man trying hard to succeed as a freelance photographer.

"She talked me into it. I was panicked that I'd never be able to handle it. Everything connected with having children loomed up as one massive unknown."

Other men respond cautiously, as did Seth and Kevin, for opposite reasons.

Seth, highly successful in an advertising career, hides a sensitive nature behind energetic, rapid-fire responses.

"I didn't dare to hope. After four miscarriages we didn't want to get too excited. I exaggerated nonchalance, for fear of breaking the spell. The reality seemed too fragile."

Kevin, who sells insurance and appears slick and sophisticated on the surface, was ambivalent underneath. He spoke thoughtfully, remembering.

"After we'd originally decided to have a baby, we got cold feet, thought maybe we should think this through a little longer. Then suddenly, quite unexpectedly, she was pregnant. I had counted on that extra time to adjust one hundred percent toward the thing."

Even an unplanned pregnancy can produce excitement. Pat, a muscular, handsome construction worker with a shock of black hair, had just married for the second time. He shook his head as he remarked, "I definitely hadn't figured on a baby. So I was surprised to find that not all my feelings were negative. Everything seemed sharper, more colorful, more alive."

Some men feel numb, apparently uninterested. While such neutrality may suggest a lack of feelings, it is usually a cover-up for emotions too strong to be recognized or dealt with. Acknowledging intense feelings can seem overwhelming, and coping with them too much to handle. Hank, a balding, slender, self-contained man who runs his own contracting business, was an example of the expectant father who protects himself by remaining at an emotional distance.

"I was detached. Disconnected. Like I had switched into neutral. I acknowledged the fact of the pregnancy and discussed it sensibly. But emotionally I was out in left field."

Following their initial reactions, most men are bombarded by a hail of positive and negative feelings. Thoughts frequently race in all directions as a fuller realization of what lies ahead hits home. Mood swings, usually associated with expectant mothers, are common among expectant fathers, too.

"You could say I felt like a tossed salad. I ran through every feeling in the book," was the way Scott, the struggling photographer, described himself.

"I was like a yo-yo, up one minute, down the next," explained the musician, Craig. "My wife's moodiness was explainable—hormones. Or so I'm told. Mine just made me feel neurotic."

Mixed emotions are an appropriate response to change, but they can be upsetting, especially when some feelings seem unsuitable for an expectant father. Some men, for example, interpret the hollow feeling that hits when pregnancy is certain as doubt about wanting the baby. Others, seeing pregnancy as an intrusion in their lives, are troubled by resentment.

For Kevin, the insurance agent, the reality of pregnancy was a worrisome blessing.

> "My ambivalence surprised me. Though I was truly looking forward to being a father, I realized I didn't want my life to change. I liked it the way it was."

"The responsibility knocked me out," admitted Pat, often weary from long days on the construction site. "Bills, a pregnant wife to care for, a child to raise. I was uneasy, irritable, generally difficult to have around."

When emotions seem inappropriate even though they are not, self-deprecation and guilt may be added to the mix.

"I felt guilty over being such a wet blanket, embarrassed at not being able to master my feelings. Feeling out of control in this way was a new experience for me," said Hank, who has his contracting business firmly in hand.

The man who has just learned that he has fathered a child faces many changes—his future plans, his relationship with his wife, the way he relates with, and is seen by, all the other people that he knows, the way he sees himself. What a cacophony of new feelings this has to produce! Yet, so universal and persuasive is the characterization of men as emotionally "cool" that many expect themselves to be just that.

This battery of confusing, disturbing emotions can produce a sense of loneliness and isolation, particularly when a man believes that he must keep such feelings to himself. Kevin, whose job demands confident, ready answers, said:

> "I wasn't nearly as exhilarated as she was. There wasn't anyone I could commiserate with. I was afraid of being seen as inadequate, which I certainly felt."

To add to the expectant father's dilemma, the confusion caused by these mixed feelings seems to interfere with gaining a solid emotional foothold. But becoming scared and doubtful, and even angry, in response to change is normal and healthy. The self-examination triggered by conflict is a necessary step within the process of coming to terms with new issues.

Every newly expectant father needs to give himself room for emotional responses that reflect the fact that the world as he knows it has just shifted under his feet. Flexibility, self-acceptance, and curiosity can help him to embrace his future fatherhood free of self-censorship, ready for change.

Clarence, the lighting engineer, dropped down from his cloud after a period of contemplation for a clear look at the future.

> "As much as we were going to have to change our lives for the baby, my greatest concern was how we could do what we do, be who we are, integrate the baby into our lives—and not just gear ourselves to the baby. I really wanted to find a point where everybody was in harmony."

Jordan, an established art dealer, was accustomed to running his business and his life with precision and order.

Now, as he looked forward to fatherhood, he summarized his feelings regarding the inevitable changes that would affect his life.

> "It's a big thing, having a baby. It changes every aspect of your life—go down the list. It takes time to adjust to each change and you must go through all of them. But I feel ready for it."

2 Changes

Planning to be a father is one thing. Feeling like a father is another. As Jordan emphasized, becoming a father is one of the most dramatic shifts of a lifetime.

Unlike expectant mothers, who usually can conjure up images of themselves caring for a new baby, expectant fathers generally have more difficulty imagining their role as fathers. Considering the prevailing attitude toward fathering in the past, this uncertainty is understandable.

Little girls play at being mothers and receive strong messages about mothering as they grow up. Mothers and daughters, and women friends, exchange information on motherhood. The games and communications of boyhood, on the other hand, are centered on career possibilities, seldom on fatherhood. Traditionally, information on fathering has not been handed down from father to son nor exchanged among men. The overall message is that fathering is not essential in defining manhood. Limitations imposed by this orientation often come as a surprise to expectant fathers.

Consider Seth, for example. Once he felt secure in acknowledging his pregnancy, he realized suddenly how limited was his knowledge of babies.

"All at once I started seeing them everywhere. But they seemed to me like helpless little outer-space creatures. If I were left alone with one, I wouldn't know what to do first."

Because men generally are so seldom exposed to babies, many expectant fathers skip over infancy in their imaginings of the future, picturing themselves instead with small children.

"I saw my child as someone I could take places, talk with about things important to me. I often imagined the two of us fishing or paddling down the river in the early morning," disclosed Eric, whose complexion was ruddy from the time he spent outdoors.

Picturing themselves with a child leads expectant fathers, and mothers as well, to resurrect their own childhoods. Memories from the past, evaluation of their own parents, strongly influence the intentions of future parents. Those whose upbringings were secure and satisfying have an advantage. They enter parenthood with minimal qualms about the outcome. But criticism is more prevalent than praise, perhaps because people tend to anticipate their own parenthood idealistically.

Andre, who cherished the image of himself as a father, found himself reviewing unhappy childhood memories with an eye to improving upon the past.

> "My father worked hard, buried himself in the paper evenings, carved the roast at Sunday dinner. We went to a ball game now and then, but I didn't really know him. He was basically a figurehead. I think I can come up with better ideas on how to relate to my child by being more conscious of who I am and how I feel."

Craig, whose kind eyes appeared slightly enlarged behind the lenses of horn-rimmed glasses, had missed being close to his father. He spoke with a mixture of sorrow and resentment.

"My father wasn't openly affectionate. He must have
loved me but he never spoke it. To this day we are
very stand-offish when we greet each other—a hand-
shake, a clap on the shoulder. God forbid a hug! I
wanted to take fathering further. I don't see myself as
less of a man if I kiss my child, or tell him that I love
him, whatever age he is."

The circumstances of raising children have changed
dramatically in recent years. With so many mothers working
outside the home, baby care and household tasks are no
longer off limits to men. This situation has served to give
men a fresh look at their fathering roles. Many have become
modern pioneers, refusing to be boxed in by traditional images of fathers solely as breadwinners, teachers, and discipli-
narians. Instead, they want to join in nurturing their children. They want to go beyond the basics of child care to
enjoy the freedom women have always had to demonstrate
love openly for their children, cuddling and caressing them,
speaking gently and tenderly in ways long seen as "feminine."

Somewhere along the way, a man anticipating fatherhood goes beyond gripes and grudges toward his own father to realize that the two of them now have something
significant in common: parenthood. Often this link leads to
a new understanding between generations that may ease
old tensions and forge new bonds.

That was Kevin's experience, to his happy surprise.
"My dad and I used to disagree on almost everything.
When he knew I was going to be a father, he started mel-
lowing out. He must have felt like this was symbolic of my
growing up, joining the ranks. For my part, I began to appreciate the responsibility of taking on a family. He worked
hard all his life to support us. I don't think I had fully appreciated that."

As male and female parenting roles overlap, the need for a couple to harmonize values and viewpoints is highlighted. Joint baby care can magnify differences of opinion, setting off discussion and sometimes heated debates—whether or not to pick up a crying baby, for example, or the virtues of cloth versus disposable diapers, or whether feeding schedules should be set by parents or baby.

When Clarence and his wife talked over the future one night after dinner, they glimpsed the importance of teamwork.

"Broadly speaking, we were in agreement. Not so with specifics. It was a jolt to realize how differently we saw certain things, and how important the differences were—like the kid's entire mental health depended on whether he should sleep alone or with us."

As men consider fatherhood, they begin to realize that they will never see themselves the same way again. As Jordan put it, "I had surrendered to the commitment, but I didn't know yet whether the reality would be positive or negative."

A primary source of anxiety is the impossibility of foretelling what many of the changes will be or how they will affect a man. Worries are sometimes easier to deal with when they are translated into questions. The practical issues can be sorted out and answered, at least in part, through reading and talking with experienced people who are able to provide factual responses to questions like: Will my wife come through labor and birth in good health? Will the child be born without defects? Which are best, doctors or midwives? Where should we have the baby?

However, it is those questions that cannot be answered in advance that seem to produce ulcers, night sweats, and migraines, as these fathers remember:

"Would my relationship with my wife change? A guy on the job warned me to make the most of what we have now because she would be a different person after the baby came. That really shook me up."

"Would a baby get in the way of my career? I was just starting as a musician—which meant very lean pickings at times. I worried that I would have to cancel out my dream in order to bring in enough steady money."

"I wondered how a baby would influence our friend-ships. Most of the people I knew had no children. The probability that we'd see less of these friends, moving off in different directions, was upsetting."

"Just exactly how would a baby tie us down? I like to take off with my wife on the spur of the moment, when the notion strikes."

"I had nightmares about not being able to find work. Although my wife had a career and was going to con-tinue to work, I saw myself as the chief means of sup-port."

"Would I have what it takes to be a good father? I had always figured that I had my good and bad points and hadn't worried much about either. But I couldn't look at myself so casually any more. What if I blew it?"

"Would I like being a father? What if I didn't like my kid? Would he love, or even like me?"

"Will our baby be normal?"

"When would I *feel* like a father?"

These kinds of questions are cliff-hangers because they are about future events or intangible issues, not concrete problems that lend themselves to immediate solutions. An expectant father can track down facts and useful predictions about physical welfare, baby equipment, or medical costs, but only time can reveal how a baby will affect a relationship, curtail independence, or change a person. Sometimes even the questions are not clear. A prospective father may simply feel a prickly sense of uncertainty about a fuzzy future, like one man who said, "Sometimes it was hard to know what we were talking about. How can you discuss what you don't know? You can't make it up!" Realizing that other expectant fathers have sweated over these intangibles and survived can lessen a man's sense of isolation and raise the odds that he will, too.

Probably the most helpful factor in assessing the future is self-knowledge. A man can ask himself how he has met the unknown in the past, what inner resources got him through successfully, and what personal traits stood in his way.

For example, one expectant father was so worried about the effect a baby might have on his marriage that he blurted out the question in class, not five minutes after he walked through the door for the first time. As we talked, it turned out that his relationship had already weathered two major challenges. He had supported his wife while she completed college, and she had managed alone when he served in the army. Each of them had grown and changed during these periods. The challenges had improved their relationship. This man had taken these successes as a matter of course, not recognizing their value as resources and reassurance for his future as a father.

Anticipating fatherhood raises legitimate questions about relationships with one's child, career, enough money to make it through, a personal life that remains intact, continuing closeness with one's wife. Waiting for answers is far from easy. The nine months of pregnancy can seem interminable—but they are also an opportunity for reflection and introspection, a chance for a man to get to know himself. "It is a bridge of time that allows you to make the emotional transition to parenthood," said Kevin.

The Physical Transformations of Pregnancy

In early pregnancy, only the slight rounding of a pregnant woman's abdomen and fuller breasts testify to a baby's presence. As Andre confirmed, at this point the pregnancy seems almost a dream. During the last months, when a woman's belly has swollen to the size of a beach ball, firm as a drum, its surface marbled in blue and rose, the visible transformation is mind-boggling.

For expectant fathers, the physical changes in the women they love produce a wide range of reactions.

"I was awed by the capacity of my wife's body to cradle a new life. She seemed like Mother Earth and a Playboy goddess rolled into one. I adored looking at her and felt tremendously tender and protective towards her."

"Neither she nor I could fully absorb the change. She would stand, naked, before the mirror, staring at herself, saying, 'This can't be me!' I've seen pregnant women but not next to me in bed. I couldn't imagine a body doing that."

"She was getting more and more tremendous by the day, yet it wasn't real to me. Her appearance was so different, she seemed like a stranger at times. She even felt different to touch. I was quite put off, which was distressing for both of us."

"Near the end she made me think of a great beached whale, resting in the middle of our bed. Her belly seemed like an extension that had nothing to do with her, leading the way as she walked about, knocking into things."

"I would look at her, touch her, communicate with her belly a lot, taking pictures of her belly, talking to the baby. That's how I got comfortable with it."

This form is vastly different from the one a woman's partner has known so well. In a society that limits female beauty to a streamlined figure, a full and rounded shape may unsettle some men. Hank's eyes twinkled, though his face remained serious, as he emphatically proclaimed his reaction: "I definitely saw her as getting fat. F-A-T!"

Generally, it is women who, comparing themselves unfavorably to fashion magazine models, view themselves as fat. Many men have a different concept of attractiveness during pregnancy. Unlike Hank, who was alienated by pregnancy's physical realities, Clarence and Craig focused on aspects of womanhood unconnected with weight gain, and found pregnant women beautiful.

Said Clarence, "Pregnant women in general, my wife in particular, turn me on. I have never seen a woman's complexion get more radiant, eyes get more bright. There's even a quality about the skin, the body—a glow. It's the highlight of the pregnant look, like beaming all over. I take pleasure in that."

Craig added, "I had difficulty understanding her feeling unattractive because I saw her as very attractive. The only time my wife wasn't attractive to me was when she herself really didn't feel attractive and didn't take care of herself as a result. What was on the inside projected to the outside."

Between the third and the fifth months, when a mother and father first can hear a tiny heartbeat and feel the baby move, pregnancy takes on another dimension. The baby's first kicks suddenly make the pregnancy real. "It was time to be serious about all those physical changes," declared one father. "This wasn't just fat after all."

At this point, the baby is completely formed, a miniature human being around 12 inches long, weighing about a pound. These first perceptible signs of life often elicit fascination, amusement, reverence. Andre, for whom the earlier absence of proof had been disconcerting, was enthralled.

"I felt like I had a relationship with this baby before it was born because I was seeing, week by week, what was physically going on. The first time you feel and see that baby move, the first time you realize that there's a little human being an inch or so beneath your hand, it's pretty incredible that there's something alive in there. I put it on videotape so we could always see that rippling."

Not all expectant fathers are equally entranced. Some men, although pleased and proud as they anticipate fatherhood, find that in their imaginations, their future child has no connection with the movements they feel. "Feeling the baby move repelled me. It was like a living parasite," said one.

Kevin had another reaction. "For me, the baby is a fetus, for my wife more of a baby. It's alive and moving, but like a tadpole, not yet a frog. To be a baby, it has to do certain things and have certain features."

Incapable of sharing in the physical development of a child, able only to look on, at times expectant fathers become envious of their wives. "At times I was jealous, feeling quite boring and ordinary next to her magnificence," stated one man who had achieved extraordinary heights in his career, yet saw pregnancy as a feat beyond compare. "I even dreamed that I was pregnant."

Envy of pregnancy or insecurity about approaching fatherhood often opens a Pandora's box of guilt and embarrassment. Such emotions can be difficult for an expectant father to handle, especially if he sees them as inappropriate for a male. One reaction, common among expectant fathers but seldom discussed or taken seriously, is the development of symptoms usually associated with pregnancy: weight gain, backache, toothache, nausea, vomiting, appetite loss, indigestion, diarrhea, constipation, leg cramps, sleep disturbances, dizziness, tension, fatigue, depression, and general irritability.

This response is known as the *couvade syndrome*, thought to be a physical response to the emotional conflicts regarding pregnancy. The word *couvade* comes from a French verb meaning "to brood" or "to hatch." Couvade syndrome differs from the couvade ritual practiced in some cultures, wherein fathers *pretend* to have symptoms related to pregnancy as part of a traditional response to pregnancy or labor. The symptoms of the couvade syndrome, which one out of ten men may experience, are very real, as some of the men we have met discovered.

"I wasn't conscious of eating more, but I gained more weight than my wife. My mind was like a sieve, and I had trouble sleeping. My life hadn't changed except for the pregnancy," said Seth.

Craig disclosed, "I used to fall into bed exhausted. Foods that never gave me trouble before caused terrific indigestion. You don't imagine heartburn."

Pat added, "When my wife complained that her back hurt, mine began bothering me, too. And terrific headaches kept me home from work. After the baby was born, I was fine."

These physical reactions can be a way of sharing in the creative experience of pregnancy, forever off-bounds to men. Symptoms usually begin around the third month and disappear as soon as the baby arrives. They may differ from the woman's symptoms or be the same, differing only in degree.

Much to his chagrin, Kevin found that it is even possible for a man to do all the suffering, while his wife sails through the pregnancy feeling wonderful.

"For three months I would wake up in the morning sick to my stomach when my secretary was pregnant and, later, with my wife's pregnancy. It would take me until about eleven o'clock until I could get going. It was a big joke because my wife felt fine. I'd tell her, 'I'm taking over your morning sickness for you.'"

Expectant fathers' reactions to this explanation of their physical woes vary. Some deny negative emotions altogether. Others readily admit worries and conflicts, but see no link between feelings and symptoms. Those who do connect the two sometimes find that symptoms magically disappear.

Our society laughs about fathers-to-be who "act pregnant." Humor (as opposed to ridicule) can lighten difficult times, but the couvade syndrome should be taken seriously. It illustrates that men, far from being emotional bystanders during pregnancy, are powerfully and intricately involved.

Partly because feelings about having a baby may be too strong to be comfortably acknowledged, and partly because fatherhood is so far in the future and seems more abstract than real, some men have a sense of neutrality toward their pregnancies.

The immediacy of a pregnant woman's physical changes, impossible to ignore, offers expectant fathers an opportunity to acknowledge emotional responses to the pregnancy that they might otherwise push aside. By acknowledging their reactions to physical changes, they may become aware of other emotions related to having a child. Eric, barely twenty years old, was among many fathers of all ages who said they learned to know themselves more fully by being open to all that they were feeling. He recalled:

> "You see her getting bigger and bigger, and you know your life is changing. You start to wonder what *you're* doing that's interesting and productive. You're stopped short when it hits you that the girl you married is really a woman. Then you start thinking about yourself as a father—and you take a giant leap away from child-hood."

A Changing Relationship

Imagine a man and a woman living harmoniously together. One day a third person, of great importance but totally unfamiliar and completely helpless as well, comes to live with them—permanently! Overnight, their lives are changed.

Even before their baby is born, expectant parents find their relationship with one another affected. All at once stability is a paramount concern. Exactly how solid is their union? Simon, an earnest young lawyer, found himself giving serious thought to the values and priorities that characterized his partnership with his wife.

"We were more conscious of flaws, fragilities that might turn out to be terminal, splitting us up. No future for a baby."

Such scrutiny can magnify previously insignificant personal traits into major issues. Wearing steel-rimmed glasses that emphasize his thoughtful nature, Simon recalled his observations.

"With my wife everything has to be perfect. The slightest little thing will throw her into a tailspin. Also, she's a worrier and when she worries, she picks. How was she going to handle being a mother? But she gets such a kick out of babies. And she's great at communicating with kids. That was in her favor."

A pregnant woman, preparing for motherhood, also goes through some soul-searching. Temporarily, she is likely to become uncharacteristically introverted. Nicholas, who, as a social worker, was trained to be objective about people's behavior, was no different from many expectant fathers when he became puzzled and upset by his wife's changed personality.

"I thought I knew her pretty well. Suddenly, there she was, keeping to herself with this one-track mind about pregnancy. Being so self-centered was out of character for her. I went through hard times convincing myself that things had not soured between us."

The mood swings of a pregnant woman can be abrupt and extreme. Like other men, Nicholas found it difficult to remain objective as he wondered whether he was the cause of trouble in his once-predictable relationship.

"Things of little consequence made her furious, like my forgetting to bring home salad greens for dinner. In the middle of an argument, she could go from crying to laughing within seconds. I felt I was walking a tight-rope, trying to figure out what I'd done this time, how to respond."

Kevin described himself as impatient and skeptical. "All these changes! You've been living with this lady for so long, and all of a sudden she's acting like a different person. My attitude was, 'Come on, it's like a cold. It'll get better.' I didn't appreciate what she was going through."

Hank became annoyed. "I think her anxiety infected me, though I covered it over by kidding. She read books *ad nauseum*, libraries full, almost overdoing it."

A pregnant woman, undergoing a revolution in every cell of her body, looking ahead to one of the major physical challenges of her life, needs support. Her husband, the future father, is the obvious candidate. But because he is a man and not physically involved, he may view the upcoming birth less emotionally than his wife does, and possibly may lack some of the sympathy she needs. Although Clarence had a compassionate, perceptive nature, he found that trying to understand his wife was a tough assignment.

"Sometimes I tried to imagine myself reincarnated as a woman, with my man's mentality, so I could fully appreciate what she was going through. It was especially difficult when she would get into her crying routine, saying I didn't understand. I didn't, and it was frustrating."

A woman is not alone in reacting to the pressures of pregnancy. An expectant father experiences his own inner turmoil. As he struggles with the changes in his wife, the responsibilities he faces, the search to see himself as a parent, his behavior changes, too. Many expectant fathers share similar reactions:

"Sometimes, like on New Year's Eve, she didn't want to go out. But me, I really wanted to party. Of course we didn't, and I felt angry about that, putting aside my own wishes, even though I tried to understand."

"I know that I was less present for her than she needed me to be. This bothered me a lot, but I felt incapable of changing it. I was caught up in the need for quiet and solitude, my own thinking time."

"Money! If you have it, you feel good about yourself. If you don't, your self-esteem is not so hot. We were irritable with each other because we were frightened that we hadn't saved enough to have a baby—even though we knew that, if we'd planned it, we never would have had a kid because we never would have been perfectly ready."

"Midway into pregnancy I became impotent. In no way had I lost interest in sex. I think I was scared about what we were heading into, and whether I could take it all on."

Lovemaking

When a couple's relationship is stressed, lovemaking is one way to smooth over the rough edges, re-establishing affection, intimacy, desirability. But this source of reassurance is not always available to expectant parents. Although lovemaking increases for some couples during pregnancy, and remains the same for others, for the majority there is a gradual decrease, with little or no intercourse by the ninth month.

Scott's anxiety about becoming a father, which caused him to become impotent, is one example of how a man's emotions can interfere with his sexual responses.

Andre, on the other hand, was delighted with his sex life during pregnancy:

> "She became extremely tender and passionate toward me when she was pregnant. And since it was the baby, at least indirectly, who brought on these changes I felt pretty good toward him, too."

Simon's situation was more typical. "Morning sickness and feeling tired—she slept all the time—put the lid on everything at first. After that passed and she felt good again, our sex life more or less went back to normal. But as she got further into pregnancy, big and uncomfortable, she became less interested in sex, which made sense to me."

Contrary to the common notion that women dictate the sexual schedule during pregnancy, expectant fathers' reactions contribute equally to changes. Jordan, nearly forty, had absorbed himself totally in the experience of becoming a father. Fascinated, he thoughtfully considered each new development.

"I felt that in some way pregnancy itself may give off some kind of chemical that reduces a man's sexual urge. I found that my sexual feelings diminished—not my love, just my sexual drive—as the pregnancy came more into bloom."

Hank was affected by his wife's personality changes.

"I was very upset because I had trouble being aroused by my wife. I couldn't come to terms with the *very* serious person she was becoming."

Many men respond to the pregnant form with appreciation and pleasure—"I loved caressing her. She felt delicious, like a ripe peach"—but others are turned off. One expectant father expressed the feelings of several others when he said, "I had expected problems with my ability to relate to her on a physical level." What he hadn't anticipated was that he "was unable to ignore my feelings to the extent that I assumed I would be able to." Some men are upset by the way a pregnant woman's skin feels, cells filled with extra fluid. Increased vaginal secretions, with a different aroma and taste, can inhibit sex. A greatly rounded abdomen makes a number of positions difficult or even impossible. Enlarged breasts may be painfully, rather than erotically, sensitive. Hank felt guilty and anxious about his reaction to his wife.

"The pregnant shape isn't sexy to my way of thinking. There's too much of everything. I prefer the long, lean way my wife used to look. I imagined her never looking that way again."

For expectant mothers, too, the pregnant image influences libido. Many women see themselves as fat—a view all too often thoughtlessly seconded by their doctors. Especially if a woman doubts her attractiveness and sexual appeal, her husband's opinion will be crucial to making her feel sexually desirable. "Sometimes I became impatient because nothing I said made any difference," complained one husband.

Tucked away in the subconscious of some men, there is a notion that having and enjoying sexual urges toward a pregnant woman is unacceptable, even sinful. "I had this kind of reverence for her," Nicholas was surprised to discover. "There were times when I found her desirable but I couldn't follow through, particularly as the baby began to show. She was like a madonna, off-bounds." After a thoughtful pause he came right to the point: "You don't go to bed with mother!"

Ardor cools when men worry that intercourse might cause physical harm to their wives or babies. While real risk can be determined only by a doctor, the developing infant is normally quite safe, immersed in fluid behind the tough, resilient muscle barriers of the mother's abdominal wall, uterus, and cervix. An expectant father's undue concern can extend to himself, contributing to impotence, as it did with Scott.

> "I felt exposed and vulnerable when I was inside, imagining the baby just a few inches away. I had this idea that I might get bitten. Maintaining an erection became a problem."

For some men, the baby's presence can enhance the sexual atmosphere. One father observed, "At times the pregnancy was the reason for our lovemaking. Sex took on a special intimacy, became real *love*-making."

Andre's experience was similar: "My fascination with the baby's movements, stroking my wife's round smooth belly, often led to lovemaking. We took more time than usual, explored each other more slowly and sensually. I felt extraordinarily open with her."

Other men, Kevin among them, find that feeling and observing the new life interrupts intimacy.

"The baby's presence was unavoidably obvious toward the end—great thumping kicks and somersaults. We carried on, but I found the movements distracting. It was too basic. I prefer sex to be less primitive, more mysterious."

Men say that going without sex for long periods during pregnancy means more than the absence of orgasm.

"Aside from the physical frustration, which I could relieve somewhat through masturbation, I missed the intimacy," Clarence commented. "The loss of this kind of closeness became a strain on us both. Everything mounts up, all the minor difficulties, and this ties a ribbon on the package."

Relationships can be further strained when expectant fathers accompany their wives to medical checkups and observe vaginal exams. Pat and Scott reported:

"After the first one I came out thinking, 'I never saw another man touch my wife.' I was definitely jealous and angry at the doctor. I wanted to punch him out."

"I was uncomfortable, thinking that it might hurt her and that she might be embarrassed to have me looking on while she was exposed."

For Simon, the visits were "pretty clinical. Instead of seeing him as fooling around with my wife I chose to see it as making sure that she would be all right. I figured this was his job."

Often, a man's outward response to stress is intellectual, whereas women react on an emotional level. As a result, women sometimes complain about missing emotional connections with men, while men believe women are overreacting when they permit their feelings to show. In fact, behind a cool exterior, a man can be seething. Seth told of his reaction to advice on sex during pregnancy:

"We had heard so many tales of what we could or could not do, we began to feel like guinea pigs. Finally we threw away the books and experimented with what suited us. The research was very stimulating."

When sex, or certain aspects of it, are put on hold during pregnancy, the absence of physical intimacy must be countered by other expressions of affection. Communication is vital to keeping a man and a woman from erecting barricades between one another, especially when new needs may leave the couple floundering, out of touch at times. Deeply personal discussions were difficult for Pat and his wife to initiate, even harder to sustain.

"We always had a good scene in bed but didn't talk about it. Things changed so much during pregnancy that we *had* to talk or else turn into strangers. We did it somehow. Keeping in mind that we love each other cut through a lot of baloney."

Hank was less given to introspection.

"I had never been one to discuss our relationship, and it was like pulling teeth to get me into it. But for us it was essential. If we avoided the issues, they built and built to the point where it seriously threatened us. We talked together, which wasn't always harmonious. Knowing that I was worried increased her worries, on the one hand, but getting things out into the open allowed us to work for solutions."

Because lovemaking is such a personal aspect of a couple's relationship, the consternation caused by unexpected changes during pregnancy is often kept private. Expectant parents need to keep in mind that it is normal to be tuned in to each other at times and to be out of sync at others.

Fortunately, a number of younger men report, couples are less hesitant to reach beyond themselves for understanding and direction than they once were. Sharing experiences with other expectant parents, perhaps friends or couples met at pregnancy classes, can be enormously reassuring.

Time alone is important, too, a temporary respite from the pressures of a relationship in flux. Clarence found this helped to restore his inner sense of self.

"Some nights I couldn't wait for her to go to bed. Which didn't mean I didn't love her. She's pregnant, you're trying to be the perfect husband, and occasionally you just want time to be by yourself. I'd sit up, watch TV, and sleep on the couch. It did make bad feelings between us, and on the surface I felt guilty about enjoying my own space—but way down inside, no."

For some men, the need for private space may expand into a more generalized withdrawal, self-protection rather than self-restoration. For these men, it may seem easier, less threatening, to distance themselves from the pregnancy than to try to deal with their feelings. Some men absent themselves from home at critical times—like one expectant father who insisted he couldn't miss an out-of-town business convention scheduled for the week his wife was due to give birth.

Even though pregnancy-related changes are temporary, expectant fathers are often uncomfortably aware that the changes are beyond their control. For some men an extra-marital fling, usually brief and superficial, offers temporary reassurance. So confessed a long-haul trucker named Charlie, a gruff, serious man who, throughout the pregnancy, had been uncertain of his importance to his wife.

> "Sex outside was something I had thought of but never actually considered seriously. I really didn't want anyone else. During the pregnancy a couple of one-night stands eased the tension and reminded me that I was a man, but I'm not sure the guilt was worth it."

Distance may make some men feel safer, but it risks weakening relationships. The man who elects to involve himself and to remain open to his feelings will do best if he allows emotions to surface without self-condemnation. Choosing to adjust to circumstances rather than to struggle against them can restore a sense of control. After a lot of soul-searching, Pat came to feel that he was more at ease getting into his feelings than circling around them. "That don't-let-your-guard-down stuff is strictly for robots," he announced.

Other fathers made these observations:

"Especially during the last two to three months, sexually and socially, my life changed. I didn't like it. I wasn't able to make peace with it. But I could accept it by telling myself that's how it is for now. There's nothing I could do about it on her end, so the change would have to come from my end. It wasn't easy, but in spite of a lot of strife I never worried that our relationship was in question."

"If I could get going, feel better about myself, then she could feel a little better about what she was going through. She felt the strength in me. It didn't work all the time, but it worked when it worked."

"Sometimes both of us were so aware that electricity was in the air, we simply tried to stay out of each other's way. Getting heated over insignificant things took its toll. Whatever it was would work out when we were able to let it be a little."

The goals, as these fathers saw them, are to be open and clear in exchanging requests for support with their mates and in explaining what is needed, to share experiences, but to allow each other space and privacy as well, to respect each other's differences. Ultimately, the differences round out a relationship. As Jordan noted:

"Our relationship is stronger, more solidly grounded than before. We are less complacent and casual, more appreciative of the reasons we care about each other. It took a lot of work. You can't live on moonlight and roses forever. Becoming parents was welcome to us. The unity of purpose channeled our energies, bonding us more closely. It is friendship deepening."

Nurturing Expectant Fathers

"Nurturing" is a word that pops up regularly in conversations about pregnancy. "Women need nurturing when they're pregnant." "Midwives are more nurturing than doctors." "Fathers want to join their wives in nurturing their children."

What is being said here? Nurturing is a vital element of human interaction. It is caring that comes from the heart, a loving effort to help someone weather difficult times in ways that bolster confidence and self-sufficiency, strengthen emotional security, and promote inner growth.

A pregnant woman, assaulted by physical changes, roller-coaster mood swings, and the anticipation of giving birth, needs this kind of support. But what about her husband? As co-creator of the pregnancy, mate to a pregnant woman, metamorphosing father, future partner in the raising of a child, he has unique emotional needs, too.

Yet relatives, friends, and even strangers usually are interested only in the mother. It is she who is counseled, pampered, praised. Charlie observed:

> "Not one soul, not even my parents, asked after *me*. Questions were always about my wife. She was like a queen bee, while I hung out in the background as part of the scenery. In retrospect, I can't say I liked it but I didn't think to question it."

Expectant fathers tend to be relegated to the sidelines, their needs overlooked. For example, the newfound intimacy that a man may feel for his wife as they create a child together might go unheeded by his comrades, who discuss the pregnancy in ways that praise masculine fertility and mourn loss of freedom. Such was the case with Pat, who explained, "Some of the fellows at work kidded me like I was a champion stud. Outwardly I laughed it off. Inwardly I felt isolated. I no longer saw myself as part of that type of horseplay."

Expectant fathers are often excluded from woman-to-woman trading of experiences and advice on pregnancy and birth, and from events and decisions that they might prefer to be sharing with their wives. Clarence, for one, recalled:

> "My biggest problem was with my mother-in-law saying that I wasn't taking good care of my wife. She was full of suggestions. It was like she was such an expert that my opinions didn't count. I didn't want to fight with my wife and I was afraid of offending my mother-in-law. It was a strain on me."

Then there's the obstetrician. Although many men are permitted—occasionally invited—to accompany their wives to office visits, some expectant fathers feel more like "excess baggage," as Pat put it, than equal partners in producing a baby.

> "How many times did I hear 'The doctor said. . . .' I was jealous of him, always smooth and confident, always there for her, answering her questions, telling her what to do. With me he was polite but aloof."

One of the greatest difficulties for an expectant father is his sense of being stranded, uncertain where he fits in, unclear about how to get his needs met. He is often seen as a smoothly functioning machine, presumed to suffer few emotional upheavals connected with pregnancy, the obvious person to give support.

There is no doubt that acting as helpmate to his wife—shouldering housework and errands—is appropriate and important. Aside from the obvious benefit to his wife, this gives a man a concrete part to play in the pregnancy. As Craig put it, "I felt such love for her and wanted to help in every way I could."

The drawback is that a man's importance as an expectant father may be minimized or forgotten because he is identified primarily as caretaker. Yet many a man goes along with this image. Total immersion in nurturing his wife can insulate an expectant father from his feelings, which then remain unappreciated as well as unresolved. He is sidetracked from seeking his own support. As the following comments illustrate, doing all the giving usually shoves a man's anxiety out of sight only temporarily.

"My wife always made me feel like the king of the castle. It was kind of an about-face when she became so involved in herself. I felt a bit lost."

"I enjoyed taking care of things at first, but it did begin to wear a little thin. I felt guilty that I couldn't take it in stride, but some of that special attention would have felt good to me, too."

"Her insecurity and apprehension about not knowing what was going on in her body were hard on us. I was always trying to be reassuring, while she was always thinking the worst, which I didn't understand. If I had been more tuned in to my emotions, I could have been more effectively sympathetic. It felt like a burden to have to be reassuring."

"All that husbandly mothering served to keep the lid on my own worrying, but only for a while. My worries got bigger as she got bigger."

"I realized that I had my own collection of questions and dark worries as a husband, future father—a man involved with pregnancy. There were times when I wanted to throw up my hands and walk out of the house for a while, wanted to take a step back for a minute and say, 'Hold on! I'm falling apart here.'"

Men are often unused to experiencing themselves as such emotional beings. The image doesn't fit the confident, calm masculinity that a man expects of himself, or that others expect of him.

On top of this, a man may not be certain that his feelings are appropriate. He isn't pregnant; on the other hand, it's his baby, too. It is not clear whether he can or even should try to change the emotional situation. To complicate matters, much of an expectant father's anxiety focuses on rapid change with uncertain outcome months, or even years, away instead of tangible problems that lend themselves to definitive action.

Because being on the sidelines has been traditional for expectant fathers, and full pregnancy partnership is relatively new, taking the initiative to achieve recognition and support can be difficult. There are few precedents. The father of an expectant father probably made his own way during pregnancy, enlightened mainly by time and chance. "My dad raised me to meet a challenge on my own," commented Pat.

It may seem easier for a man to pretend that nothing is wrong, to try tricks or manipulation to command attention, or simply to hope that someone—preferably his wife—will notice his needs. Generally, however, such approaches only produce further frustration and alienation. This topic brought a rush of responses from fathers:

"The guys I was spending most of my time with were not fathers, so I was the strange one. And the guys I see who have children—we go out, but we don't talk about these things. So I kept quiet and played it cool, too. My question now is, whose benefit was it for?"

"It took me several months to realize that the 'unavoidable' tasks that kept me after hours at work were things that, in the past, I always made it a point to walk out on promptly at five o'clock."

"I used to let things ride, ride, ride. I was afraid to say anything a lot of times because it was her show. *She* was pregnant. How would it look if *I* complained?"

"There were times when I just lay on the couch feeling depressed. I could have used a few strokes myself, but she never guessed, and I never asked."

Where can a man turn with his special emotions related to pregnancy? Craig was fortunate. His wife realized what he was going through and reached out to him unsolicited. He spoke earnestly as he described her response:

"I've always gotten a lot of support from my wife. I know I need it, but she is the one who sees when I start to lose it, puts me back on the right track, giving me lots of strength. She was the one who tuned in to my needing support during pregnancy. She used to remind me that I am who I am, and that the child was not going to take away from me and our life, but only enhance these."

Scott received some nurturing from his mother. Her gestures of maternal benevolence provided at least a reprieve from the demands of pregnancy. He explained, "Sitting down to my favorite foods, being fussed over and made much of, restored me to myself at least temporarily."

For Hank, being with other men helped to offset the sometimes-overwhelming atmosphere of pregnancy and baby production, giving him back his sense of self. "I began to feel engulfed by baby talk," he said. "When I stopped after work for a beer with the crew, it was like a relief."

Some of Clarence's emotions became clearer when he opened up to friends. He recalled, "I never stopped seeing my buddies. I played a good deal of golf that summer, and we would talk a lot. One friend has two kids. That helped."

Some men may be fortunate enough to find a fathers' discussion group, or bold enough to organize one. These men discuss pregnancy from a male viewpoint, in a friendly, non-judgmental atmosphere. Knowing that he is not alone in his experience is one of the most powerful ways an expectant father can receive support. Learning to talk about his feelings is a vital step toward getting the attention he needs and deserves. Kevin joined such a group, not altogether willingly, and was surprised by the results.

"The group was my wife's idea. I honestly thought I had no particular worries other than the need to know that my wife and baby would be okay. But I talked about things I hadn't even guessed were on my mind."

Every expectant father explores new territory and, because there is no map to show a starting point, has the advantage of starting wherever it feels right. In his own way, each man can become part of the creativity that surrounds his child's development. Some do this by taking advantage of special talents. Kevin remarked, "One weekend I worked out all our finances for the coming year. That was something she couldn't do, for sure. It eased our minds on that score, anyway."

Expectant fathers often experience increased energy and productivity throughout the pregnancy. Clarence remembered: "Some of the stickiest technical projects at work were a piece of cake for me."

Along with their wives, some expectant fathers make it a point to seek out midwives or those doctors who view pregnancy and birth as a family matter, involving both parents from conception on out. Craig felt he had a right to understand the care that would affect his child's growth and his wife's health. Familiarity with a subject generates confidence and promotes participation.

> "I chose to go to office visits with her to be close to her and to be a part of the whole experience. They were also an instant source of information about pregnancy and birth—which were a total mystery to me. I used to be the only guy there. That felt good, even though I came home and bitched about it."

Ignorance magnifies feelings of isolation; sharing softens them. Discussing fears lessens their power. Pregnancy is a time for couples to redefine their loyalties to one another. Hank laughed as he described how well his wife understood him.

"She used to read aloud from books on pregnancy
while we were in bed, with me a captive audience. In
spite of my resistance—I was quite determined to be a
non-participant—I became intrigued."

If an expectant father remains on the edge of his pregnancy, he is the loser, shut off from the participation that is
rightfully his. He may find himself waiting out the nine
months in limbo. The more directly he can be involved, the
sooner he will feel connected with his baby after birth, and
the more opportunities he will discover for growth and en-
richment.

Most important is how a man sees himself in relation to
the pregnancy. His role is different from his wife's, but he is
not a secondary participant. He is a teammate who can
take part in ways that truly reflect his personal needs,
wishes, and goals. As he creates his own niches in his pregnancy, he needs to respect and value his feelings. Ideally, he
will recognize that having a wide range of emotions is human, not a matter of being male or female. He is no less a
man for requiring, seeking, and accepting recognition and
emotional support for himself. Once an expectant father can
see himself as a full partner in his pregnancy, other people
in his life will start to see him that way, too.

3 Birth: Whether to Participate

In New Guinea, members of certain tribes do not realize that there is a connection between sexual intercourse and reproduction. They are knowledgeable about the particulars of birthing, however, because women labor at home attended by friends and relatives.

People in our part of the world are better informed about life's beginnings, but ever since birthing disappeared behind the fortress of hospital walls, protected by medical ritual, most people here are astonishingly innocent of related details. When a woman and a man become pregnant, suddenly and nervously they realize that they have almost no idea of what lies ahead.

Men in particular have long been strangers to this womanly function, both in and out of hospitals, traditionally keeping their distance until everything was over but the shouting. These days, education for expectant parents and their sharing of laboring and birth is dispelling some of this mystery. Although being present is now a choice—though not a requirement—for men, a number of today's fathers wouldn't dream of being anywhere else when their babies arrive. According to Eric, it seemed unnatural to be separated. "We made that baby together. We will be together to bid him welcome to the world."

Andre said, "I'm looking forward to being more involved with my child than other fathers I see. This starts with being there when she is born, not peering through the window of a hospital nursery at a cocoon held by a masked nurse."

Not all fathers are so enthusiastic. A man who knows beyond a doubt that he does not want to be present has every right to say "no." A woman in labor needs to be attended by people who are caring, concerned, and—above all—committed to being with her. There is questionable benefit to her and to her husband if he feels that being present for labor and birth will be an endurance test for him.

Scott stated flatly, "I had no desire to watch my wife give birth. To me, it is an intimate female function. I would have felt embarrassed and hugely out of place."

Kevin was less emotional about his decision. "I love my wife and am very close to her in many ways. Both of us are quite comfortable with the idea that bearing children in the company of a woman friend, rather than myself, was a more agreeable choice."

Charlie, the truck driver, was adamant. "I could see myself turning green, or worse, keeling over. The humiliation was too much to risk. I felt lightheaded just looking at photos of babies being born."

Even for the large number of fathers who choose to be with their wives for labor and birth, the decision frequently comes with a fair dose of ambivalence and mixed emotions. Some men are swayed initially by a sense of duty and a recognition of current trends. Others are motivated by compassion and concern, the wish to see their wives through the difficult task of giving birth and the need to satisfy themselves first-hand as to the welfare of their wives and babies:

> "I received the final push from friends who raved about how great it was for them. They didn't fall apart, so I figured I'd survive at least and maybe even feel the same way they did, if I was lucky."

"She wanted me to be there so I agreed to go. But I felt that I really would prefer to pace around the waiting room smoking cigarettes. The more detached I am, the safer I feel."

"My wife's safety was very much on my mind. By being there I could make sure that everything possible was done for her. And I wanted to see my baby immediately, undressed, with my own eyes, to know myself whether everything was normal."

"I felt guilty that my part had been all pleasure, starting the baby, while she had all the physical disadvantages, including giving birth. It was my responsibility to see her through it, although I wasn't at all sure how I would react."

"At first I felt I'd be more of a hindrance than a help— but birth is probably the greatest of human events. How could I miss that?"

On the down side of the decision to be present are powerful misgivings—frightening, embarrassing, alarming. Even men who feel strongly about participating wonder how they will react to the utterly new experience of labor.

"I have heard of men crying with happiness. The idea of losing it before a roomful of strangers feels like an exposure of my most private self. I'd be mortified."

"I feel squeamish at the sight of blood and all. Other guys told me, 'Everyone is freaked out by that stuff but once it's happening you'll be fine.' I didn't believe them at all, but I was willing to find out. I did warn the doctor of my nervousness."

"The thought of seeing my wife in pain terrified me. I was convinced I'd become a total vegetable and that my presence could only distract and worry her."

"I hadn't the faintest notion what would be required of me. She couldn't clue me in in advance, being equally ignorant. Could she ever forgive me—or I, myself—if she turned to me and I could only stand there like a dummy?"

"I wanted to know immediately if anything went wrong, but I worried about my reaction. Maybe I'd start punching out the doctor, yelling at him, 'Why did you let this happen?' Or I'd become a gibbering idiot."

Uncertainties can be resolved, at least in part, only through experience. But an armament of facts gathered from books and the childbirth classes that abound today can help to prepare expectant fathers for what lies ahead. A man who is inclined to absent himself from the birth out of fear or prejudice will have more confidence in a decision founded on knowledge. Even a father who is certain he won't attend will be better off equipped with facts instead of fantasies to see him through the waiting. Scott, whose wife's labor was normal and uneventful, suffered agonies because of ignorance.

"What you don't know *can* hurt you. Whenever I asked—every ten minutes?—after my wife, the nurse answered, 'Oh she's fine. It'll be several hours yet. Have another cup of coffee.' Several hours? Was that normal? Were they lying? Time dragged by. I was sick with apprehension. My imagination went wild. When they finally brought me this stranger of a baby, I felt battered, bruised with relief."

Years ago, birth preparation courses trained women only. Fathers came in for a final class to receive a digested version of the overall picture. As time went by and men joined for the entire course, they evolved from spectators into labor coaches, active participants in the birthing.

The purpose of today's childbirth classes is to replace myths about birth with facts, to explain hospital routines and medical equipment and procedures, and to teach women techniques for working with labor and birth and men how to guide and encourage their partners in using these skills.

Most hospitals, birthing centers, and home birth professionals insist that would-be coaches for labor and birth complete an approved childbirth course as a prerequisite for being present. The rules are waived occasionally but a father will feel more secure if he is informed and doesn't have to enter the labor room cold turkey.

Although expectant fathers almost always accompany their wives to childbirth classes these days, they often arrive with mixed feelings.

Pat, who spent his working days in an all-male environment, recalled, "I was put off completely by the image of a room packed with women chatting enthusiastically about birth and babies."

Hank, carefully self-protective, said, "I didn't want some evangelistic type preaching at me. I am definitely unenthusiastic about being told what to do."

Seth remembered feeling "like a first grader walking in with a graduate student. My wife was a walking encyclopedia, having spent nearly $200 on books. From what other fathers said, they were on a similar level."

Once the course is underway, fathers agree that they are reassured by the clear, precise information they receive. For many men, these meetings, usually a series of six to ten lessons taken once a week, provide their first opportunity to mingle with other expectant fathers. These fathers put their reactions into words:

> "I wanted to meet other people who were expecting. I especially wanted to talk to men about going through what I was experiencing, to affirm that I was normal."

> "I was amazed by the mechanism of the female body. To my surprise, I found explanations about birth spellbinding. A baby's development and birth are a fantastic process. Toward the end of the course I got so I didn't even mind passing up Monday night football."

On a personal level, birth classes today still are geared mainly for women, just as they were years ago. The woman is, after all, the person having the baby. But this limited focus can be a disadvantage for her partner. Simon, while deeply committed to helping his wife, pointed out somewhat resentfully that his own needs during classes were ignored:

> "Classes provided me with an intellectual understanding of the birth process and some techniques for coping with concentration—but all presented from a woman's point of view. I felt that I was expected to function without any qualms in spite of an utterly strange setting, somewhat like being on automatic pilot."

Seth, who had tempered his ebullient nature throughout the pregnancy in view of the trauma of past miscarriages, exclaimed, "I always expected natural childbirth, but it took a couple of classes before I realized *how* natural! My clinical view started to slip, and the emotional intensity of being present for the birth began to come through."

Men face unique challenges during labor in their roles as coach—diplomat, liaison, on-looker, loving friend—a combination that can't help but produce a formidable mix of responsibility and vulnerability. Classes have yet to address the issues of men's feelings regarding their participation in labor, where they can look for support while the drama unfolds, or how they can rejuvenate their own confidence and sense of self if that should become necessary.

A sensitive, skilled instructor will encourage expectant fathers and mothers to discuss their feelings, especially negative ones. Men say that talking frankly with each other gives them the opportunity to become familiar with emotions that otherwise might not surface until labor is underway, and to explore avenues of resolution together. Most important, peer support boosts self-confidence.

It may be up to the men in the class to initiate this sort of communication. As his wife became more obviously pregnant, Pat had become increasingly nervous about accompanying her in labor. Courageously, he broke the ice in his first class:

> "When the instructor asked why we had come to the course, every man replied in the same vein—to learn, to become informed, etc. I said right out that I was scared shitless. There was a burst of relieved laughter, and everyone started talking at once, comparing notes."

Fathers frequently report that being present for labor and birth is physically demanding, emotionally taxing, and tempered by doubts that hang on to the end—but the vast majority state unequivocally that attending the birth of their child is the highlight of a lifetime. If a man does not at least examine his potential for exploring new frontiers, he could lose out on an experience that is beyond compare. Andre pointed out that each child is born only once. He went on to say:

"I think the world has become a little too antiseptic. The natural processes have been removed from people. Having a baby isn't an operation, and prepared childbirth is not just a bunch of techniques for giving birth. It is an attitude about birth, about a natural thing. Approaching the experience with love and respect and honoring the two people who are creating life, and the baby as well, is an affirmation of humanity. Perhaps this can be the start of making things better not just for ourselves but for all mankind."

BIRTH

"I would say to other expectant fathers, 'Try to be as calm as you possibly can. Just be there to fill in the gaps where she needs you. Stay back when you need to stay back. If your mate needs your help, reach out and do what you are able.'"

"Having your own baby is like nothing else on earth. I have bonded with my mate and my baby and have seen their strengths and have seen the whole experience evolve and it's mine til death. That vision is with me for life."

4 Labor Begins

One day, usually somewhere between the thirty-eighth and forty-second week of pregnancy, an expectant mother will experience signs that labor is beginning: the appearance of blood from the dilating cervix, a gush of water via the vagina from the broken bag of water surrounding the baby inside the uterus, and frequent, strengthening contractions of the uterus itself. These signs may occur in any sequence, well apart from each other, close together, or even concurrently.

After waiting for so many months, perhaps after a false alarm or two in the final weeks, many prospective parents hesitate to take these first signs seriously. When it became clear to Eric that labor had truly begun, the moment was exhilarating.

> "When she quietly stated that what she was feeling had to be more then the effects of the prune juice, I was instantly on my feet, thrilled and jubilant, shouting, 'This is the day! This is the day!'"

The relative inactivity of pregnancy has now given way to action. For Nicholas, the concept of fatherhood suddenly became very real.

> "While we were standing in line at the supermarket, she whispered to me that her water was leaking. That's when it really sank in that I was going to be a father. I had no sense of urgency—just quietly elated and aware of a strong protectiveness toward my wife."

Abruptly and unavoidably, an expectant father is confronted with coping with labor. Nervousness frequently goes hand in hand with excitement and readiness for action.

"I didn't want to wake up," admitted Kevin. "When she told me, I replied, 'That's impossible. Just rub your tummy.' And, conscious only of feeling extremely tired, I rolled over and went back to sleep. Two minutes later, I sat bolt upright, realizing what she had said. In that instant, I felt overwhelmed by responsibility."

Craig recalled, "My wife was very calm and lay in bed resting. I had chest pains and was up and dressed immediately."

Seth described himself as "completely calm." He said, "I remember thinking with astonishment, 'Is this really *me*?!'"

Early labor is a period of light contractions that soften the cervix and announce themselves every fifteen to twenty minutes or thereabouts. It can be thought of as a warm-up for active labor. Although Andre's enthusiastic immersion in pregnancy and approaching fatherhood suggested utter confidence, he was sufficiently anxious to be unaware when labor began.

> "For several hours she was having light contractions. I was working in the next room, going back and forth some, and didn't notice anything. Then, friends dropped over and, after a little while, someone said to me, 'Haven't you noticed? She's in labor!' I was dumbfounded."

For a first baby, this phase usually ambles along for an average of eight to ten hours. Occasionally it spreads itself over a couple of days. Because there is no way to forecast the overall length of labor, the wisest response for parents now is to remain calm and to conserve energy.

Fathers like Hank and Craig, looking back on their experiences, adamantly advise both expectant parents to rest and, if possible, to sleep, especially when labor begins at night, as it did for Hank.

> "We made the ultimate error of sitting up all night, jovially timing contractions and playing cards with friends. By morning, as labor was becoming stronger, we were a weary crew. For my wife, especially, getting into heavy contractions, the lack of sleep was a real drag. I could have kicked myself for being so shortsighted. We had felt so festive when labor began, like starting off on a holiday, that we ignored our own good sense."

Craig's wife started having contractions one morning before breakfast. "She said it was too early for me to do anything for her. In a frenzy of nervous energy, I dove into cleaning the house. She relaxed in bed laughing."

The trick is to spend this early time in ways that allow for maximum energy conservation while keeping sufficiently occupied to avoid becoming bored or jittery. A high-gear response to contractions is unnecessary during early labor, but the teamwork between parents starts here. Working together while labor is warming up and still mild establishes a unity that carries over into stronger, more active labor later on. Sharing this prelude in quiet privacy, as these men did, promotes confidence and makes conscious relaxation easier. These qualities are invaluable in meeting the challenge to come.

> "It was a beautiful day, so we passed the early hours on cushions relaxing in the garden, keeping a record of the time between contractions. I felt very close to my wife, realizing that this was our last time alone together at our home."

"To distract her and to help us both relax, I read to her from the newspaper. It was a shot in the dark, and it worked. I felt proud for both of us. We were managing."

"The midwife said we could wait it out for a while and see what happened. So everyone sat back and relaxed. The bedroom was heated with a potbellied stove so it was nice and warm, and my sister-in-law's kids were playing with blocks and coloring. My wife would say, 'Begin,' and everyone would breathe and relax with her. It was wonderful. The environment kept me calm."

Sometimes the early phase of labor sneaks silently by, unperceived by the mother. Then, as these fathers found, the stronger contractions of active, progressive labor can come on with a flourish. Although there may be several hours yet to go before the baby arrives, the suddenness of powerful labor is sometimes disconcerting.

"Things were happening so fast I didn't know what to do first," recalls Scott. "Should I help her to dress, call the doctor, or warm up the car? I think I rushed from her to the phone to the back door and back at least three times before making up my mind." Simon remained calm. "Jubilant, with butterflies in my stomach, I wrote a note to our dinner guests, pinned it to the door, and off we went."

Pat described the last fifteen minutes at home:

"Two parts of me were in operation at the same time. One, scared, saying, 'Hurry! To the hospital!' The other, moving slowly, cool, thoughtful. 'Think! Remember what you've learned.' I told my wife just to sit there and I'd help her dress, but I was so nervous that I pulled out the drawstrings at the shoulders and then couldn't find any pins, so I tied the dress together."

Clarence looked back with frustration and triumph.

"She called me and said, 'No hurry—they're twenty-five
minutes apart.' A few minutes later, when I got home,
I began timing contractions and I said, 'We'd better get
going; they're two minutes apart.' She said, 'No, you're
doing it wrong.' So I called the doctor and told *him*
and *he* said, 'You must be doing it wrong—but come
in and we'll see.' Three hours later we had the baby."

Driving with his laboring wife to the place where their
child will be born, a man feels an immense responsibility for
their safety. Although Clarence and Pat laughed as they
recalled their trips, they agreed that the thought of giving
birth in the back seat of the car, even though it rarely happens, can trigger the urge to travel as rapidly as possible.
Clarence, who lives in the country, recalled his trip:

"I was so nervous that I must have hit every pothole
and bump along the entire route. Each time, my wife,
already sounding like a locomotive, puffed louder and
faster. The only way I could keep from speeding was to
concentrate on keeping the speedometer needle below
45 mph. When we reached the hospital, I felt like they
should have brought out *two* wheelchairs."

As a city dweller, Pat remembered:

"We ran into rush hour traffic and she did her breathing
in the taxi while I sat next to her and breathed with
her. She was amazingly nonchalant about it but the
driver looked a little frantic. I guess I was pretty dis-
traught myself because I left the suitcase in the cab and

had to shout him down while she had another contraction draped over the parking meter in front of the hospital."

Most times couples can count on reaching the hospital in plenty of time and so can move along slowly and carefully, avoiding the hazards of a wild, speeding drive. Simon described the trip as magical, a suspended interval celebrating an ending and a beginning.

"She preferred the back seat of the car with pillows propped behind her. We drove slowly and chatted between contractions. Going through the park, I remember the brilliantly blue sky, gleaming white snow on the ground, the incredible stillness, and how beautifully tranquil we both felt. The presence of life was everywhere."

5 Labor and Coaching

The opening of the female body to release the new human being, formed during pregnancy from a minuscule seed to a hefty six- to nine-pound baby, is an extraordinary phenomenon, to which fathers respond with strong emotion.

> "I was awed by the power of it, that ancient birthing process, and secretly relieved that I would never have to face the challenge. I questioned whether I, as a male, would have the dedication she did, sticking with it, totally absorbed for hours."

> "I sat on the bed so she could lean against me. I could feel her energy, the energy of labor, almost as a part of me."

> "My wife was in intense labor for many hours. The strength of her contractions shocked me. I worried about their normalcy and about my wife. There was no way classes could have prepared me for this."

The magnitude of the biological energy that widens the cervix and moves the baby through the birth canal is astonishing. Women have a reservoir of toughness and strength far more powerful than anything required in day-to-day living, which often emerges for the first time in labor, propelling them through it, sometimes with their cooperation, sometimes without it.

Textbook descriptions of labor give us prosaic facts and figures: labor is divided into three stages, dilation of the cervix, birth, and the passage of the afterbirth; the whole process takes an average of twenty hours; contractions last around sixty seconds, the intervals between them, five to one minutes. But this basic information is a far cry from the remarkable, almost overwhelming physical and emotional experience. Actual labor is a stunning leap from theory to reality.

Even the movement of time is unfamiliar. The pace of passing minutes and hours changes, as Jordan noted calmly and Seth with mounting concern, while they waited out labor's first stage. Because every labor is individual for every woman, there is no answer to the pressing question, "When will it end?" Experienced professionals may hazard an intuitive guess based on years of experience, but even a doctor would need a crystal ball to come up with a precise answer.

"Several hours would speed by unnoticed. Then, for a comparatively short time, I would think the hands of the clock had stopped. I felt outside of time, observing it. I was suspended, helping my wife."

"At times labor seemed like it would go on forever. Feeling always slightly on edge, wondering, wondering, if she was getting anywhere, when it would end, I tried not to get nuts over something I couldn't control and concentrated on staying cool and doing what I could for my wife. On some level I even forgot there was a baby. The only thing that was dependable were the hands of my watch. I could count on them to tick off the seconds, and then another contraction would be over. This trivial thing sustained me."

Labor usually accelerates gradually over a period of several hours. That is, in early labor, the uterus starts out by contracting briefly and mildly three or four times per hour. Bit by bit, contractions become longer and stronger with the uterus resting for a few minutes between each one. Eventually, with contractions coming at least every five minutes, active labor is underway. Such a steady, slow-paced increase allows parents time to adapt to the experience of labor. But just as every rule has its exceptions, some labors intensify suddenly and rapidly. This was Eric's experience. In the early hours at their birthing center his wife's labor retained the same moderate quality it had at home with everyone tucked up cozily around the wood stove. But when labor changed abruptly, his most difficult challenge was to adjust emotionally while feeling pressured to do the right thing.

"When I returned after a short bathroom break, her labor had become dramatically stronger. Half of what we'd learned in class had been wiped out in five minutes. This was a whole new ball game. It was exciting but frightening because all at once I wasn't sure of anything. I needed time, except that there wasn't time."

With labor fully underway and at its most powerful, a woman feels within her body forces of such intensity that she has no choice but to surrender herself to them. Inhibitions disappear in the face of this supremely demanding physical involvement. Clarence and Hank reacted strongly, although in diametrically opposed ways, to such bold, raw behavior in their wives.

"Anything primitive is beautiful to me. In labor, her aggression, her capacity to fight, to face things, came out. I found that becoming, very exciting."

"At first I was appalled to discover this earthy side to my wife who is ordinarily poised, manicured, well put together. She looked different than I had ever seen her, grunting, sweating, red-faced, almost animalistic. She was like a stranger."

During labor, modesty is unceremoniously banished by minimal privacy, vaginal exams, exposure during birth. Fathers report that, on the whole, they are ill at ease with such casualness only when it is in conjunction with staff members' callous disregard for their wives' feelings or their own. Embarrassment directly related to physical exposure is usually overridden by involvement with the labor.

A laboring woman, bombarded by forces that confront her constantly on every level, may become impatient, aggravated, frustrated. Because her husband is most familiar to her and most steadily at her side, he often becomes the target of her irritability. Pat, who had never entirely abandoned his reservations about accompanying his wife in labor, recalled that at first he felt insulted and resentful at being treated like the enemy.

"She started snapping at me, just as I expected she would. She said I was rubbing her back in the wrong place, actually flung my hand away, and glared at me when I spoke. So I walked out, just as I said I would. Then I did some thinking. She was the one in labor, not me. If it helped her to yell, okay. And I went back in."

A coach is his mate's back-up for requests when necessary, and runs interference for her when she can't be interrupted. Nicholas, used to acting as the facilitator in his marriage relationship, passed along messages or information to his wife when she was too self-absorbed to hear clearly what others were saying.

> "At some points the only comments that registered were mine. The nurse would suggest that she slow down her breathing. No reaction. I'd say it. Success! Mine was the familiar voice."

The relationship between a woman in labor and her coach is highly personal. When a father first begins actively coaching his laboring wife, he quickly learns that the helping role of the labor coach is distinctly separate from medical care. He is a familiar, caring person who is at her side throughout labor, present solely for her, a buffer against loneliness and insecurity. Having studied and practiced with his wife the relaxing and breathing skills she will use in labor, a coach can offer reminders, inspiration, and direction, strengthening her self-control, bolstering her confidence, keeping her going if she falters.

Without doubt, the most difficult aspect of labor for every attending father is seeing his wife in pain. Some women, like Jordan's wife, experience contractions only as tremendous pressure. He observed, "I never realized that any woman could have a baby without a whimper. She did feel the contractions for sure but she had that baby just like a kitten. It was the most natural thing I ever witnessed."

Most women, however, find the contractions of active labor painful, often greatly so. Even when men have been primed for the probability of labor pain, as Hank and Seth were, the reality is a shock.

> "Her pain was like nothing I could have imagined. There was no way to be prepared for it. The grimace and wide-eyed stare on her face scared me. My first

impression was that something was terribly wrong. At one point I thought, 'I've lost her. I'll be raising this baby alone and visiting her in a Home somewhere on Sundays.'"

"Part of me wanted to put my head down on the bed and cry with frustration and sorrow. I wished fervently that my experience of the contractions could be more than my finger on the stop watch. I would have given anything to take on her hard time myself."

The fact that he cannot experience labor for himself can be particularly frustrating to a man if his ignorance causes him uncertainty about how best to help. For Simon's wife, contractions had strengthened considerably since their ride through the park.

"Most difficult for me was not knowing what she was going through. How could I, a man, possibly imagine it? At one point I asked her how she felt. When she couldn't tell me, I had to fight the urge to give up, walk out. If I couldn't understand, I couldn't know how to respond."

Nevertheless, the coaching training pays off, as Clarence and his wife were particularly aware, when they worked with a short, fast, almost unrelentingly demanding labor.

"Breathing together in practice used to crack us up. We felt self-conscious, artificial. Labor was another story. Being in sync kept us going. When a contraction started to get the better of her, she followed my lead and together we breathed through it."

All labors are tremendously hard work. Frequently laboring women discover that making noise during contractions helps them to stay in control. This works by releasing tension and providing an additional focus outside of pain. Usually these responses are unplanned, something a woman does spontaneously. Because women traditionally have been taught by childbirth educators, nurses, and doctors to labor quietly, a father may need to adjust his expectations if his wife should prefer her own noisy responses over silence. Eric, whose wife coped so serenely when labor began, was startled when "she made moaning sounds during contractions. My instant reaction was that she was dying. When I asked what was wrong, she told me that making noise helped."

Coaching gives a father the opportunity to involve himself actively in labor. The more he feels that he is a participant, the more he will experience for himself the satisfaction of having been an essential part of his child's arrival. A major coaching task—encouragement and guidance—is a reversal of traditional male/female roles. A man needs to feel comfortable being supportive in order to work harmoniously with his mate in labor. These fathers explained how they took part:

> "I felt such intense love for her and told her so, many times. I knew she was working as hard as she had ever done, sometimes feeling she couldn't handle it and was letting me down. I wanted her to know that I loved her in spite of everything, because of everything, and mostly because she was herself."

> "I'm awkward around people who are sick or unhappy. But you can't clap a woman in labor on the back and tell her to buck up. Jokes are no good. I thought about

how she stood by me and told me I could make it during a rough period I had. That was a large part of what I did in labor, and it felt fine."

"I kept going because I knew this was what I had to do. I knew she was working hard and I knew I wanted to hang right in there and do the same thing."

"To a certain degree I had to be dispassionate toward her pain to carry on, holding off my feelings. I just concentrated on what we were doing. If I had let my own distress take over, I would have been good for nothing except hovering over her like a broody hen."

"Watching her fight against contractions, I wanted to tell her not to be afraid of what she was feeling, to breathe right into it. I wasn't the one in labor—maybe she'd knock my head off—but I gave it a shot. That's what got her through."

Much coaching guidance springs from combining a few facts with lots of trial and error. Even an experienced coach can't be sure what will prove effective. How a particular woman may react to labor is revealed only as the process unfolds. A man who can allow himself the flexibility to risk mistakes is more likely to come up with ways to help his partner. Hesitating to follow hunches only results in lost opportunities.

But how is a coach to know whether his choices are right? Results are obvious sometimes, but not always. A man can ask his wife, during a break between contractions, for her reactions to his efforts. At times, however, a laboring woman is too preoccupied to comment. Then, other than checking his ideas with a nurse or midwife, a father's only recourse is to rely on intuition in deciding what to try. Experiences with teamwork vary from couple to couple.

"During a run of particularly difficult contractions she did not speak to me at all," recalled Simon. "I had no choice but to follow my hunches. When one thing didn't work, I tried another. I got about two out of five that seemed to suit her."

"I was awed by her obvious reliance on me," Seth observed, "and by my power to affect her in a physical experience that was so obviously hers and hers only."

"We fell into a sort of give and take, like the partnership of dancing. Our closeness was inspiring," remembered Andre.

There are always moments of frustration when nothing seems to come right. Craig's anxiety, fairly constant throughout pregnancy and early labor, undermined his efforts to help his wife through her strong contractions. "I couldn't get her to relax, whatever I tried," he remembered. "Then the doctor would walk in, say a word or two, and she'd go limp. My ego was bruised, I have to admit."

A father-coach has to put his ego aside and learn from the situation. Yet, if his efforts fail to help his wife manage contractions tolerably, he can feel devastated, as Craig testified.

> "I had expected the techniques we learned in class to control the pain, so I was shocked to see my wife suffering so obviously. No crying or screaming, but I could tell. I did the breathing with her and everything else, but it didn't lighten things the way we'd hoped. I felt helpless."

In fact, Craig was so distressed that "at certain points it switched to where my wife was trying to cool *me* out. She was upset that I was upset."

Realistically, techniques are more likely to help a woman manage pain than to eliminate it. Clarence, able to adopt this broader definition, felt more positive about the results he and his wife achieved. "Sometimes she used the breathing to take her mind off the pain," he explained. "Mostly, she was very conscious of the pain and used the breathing to get through it."

Considering labor's intensity and drama, effective coaching can be amazingly simple. For Eric, it seemed to boil down to basics, repeated over and over, meeting the challenge of each contraction as it came along.

"For hours, I simply talked quietly, rubbed her head, and counted seconds whenever she had a contraction. Afterward she told me that helped a lot."

Clarence, whose experience was similar, commented, "She's stubborn, always has been. I wasn't sure she'd listen to me, but she did. I just went through the basics over and over and over."

Sometimes, like Jordan's wife, a woman will be entirely self-contained during labor, requiring no support other than what she draws from within herself. Despite his admiration, Jordan occasionally felt unimportant, without purpose, even a little resentful because "she ignored me completely during contractions, and in between she dozed off. I felt sort of stranded there with nothing to do."

Coaching can be a lonely business. In hospitals, unlike birthing centers, coaching fathers usually work alone, with only occasional help from busy nurses or the attending doctor. To some degree, this fact is dictated by the limited size of most labor rooms, and by regulations that restrict labor areas to the hospital staff and fathers. "I never even got to the bathroom. The nurses were constantly on the run and I didn't want to leave my wife alone," said Eric.

Birthing centers and a few hospitals with differently designed space and different rules encourage expectant parents to bring at least one other person to help with coaching. For Simon, a second coach was a companion, someone with whom he shared concerns and responsibilities, easing the pressure. "I could take a break, reorder my forces, get a second wind, and not feel guilty," he said.

An assistant coach who has not trained and practiced with the parents, however, or who is unfamiliar with their visions and goals can be a liability instead of an asset, despite the best of intentions. Nicholas described having his sister-in-law present.

> "She didn't know where to fit in, was too self-involved and ill at ease, and ended up being a distraction. I wanted to ask her to leave but didn't know what to say. I hadn't foreseen that coming up."

Ultimately, fathers find that managing their own reactions to labor, especially to pain, hinges on being able to accept the process. The more fully Simon could embrace the reality of labor, setting aside his intellectual desire to understand the pain, the more fully he could enter the experience feeling positive and constructive.

> "It was only when I realized that I *couldn't* share it that I was able to take some control over the situation and become helpful. I realized that we had no choice but to get on top and stay there. I consciously chose to do this."

When the first stage of labor is finally complete, with the cervix open and the baby ready to move down the birth canal, the sense of being in limbo is dispelled. Waiting gives way to action. The atmosphere surrounding the laboring couple is transformed. Impatience and anxiety are replaced by relief and excitement. Energy is miraculously renewed. For Eric, there was cause to celebrate.

"For me, that was the magic point in labor. There was a reason for those powerfully hard contractions. My wife was focused, not on the pain any more, but on her efforts to get the baby out."

The Unexpected

For some couples, the course of labor is unexpectedly re-routed.

"We never considered the possibility of a cesarean. That happened to other people. When the doctor announced his decision, the shock went right through me," said Hank.

The unexpected in labor usually is related to problems with the baby or mother's well-being, or to variations in the mother's physiology—the size or shape of her pelvis, or the behavior of her uterus—that interfere with the progress of labor. It also includes the medical management of these difficulties via medication, surgery, or the use of technologies like fetal monitors or x-rays. In Hank's case, the baby's position made descent through the pelvis impossible.

Although an expectant father may have been briefed in class for medical intervention during labor, detours from the expected require major emotional adjustments, worried as he is over his wife and child, perplexed over medical processes he may not fully understand, jolted by the loss of an experience he envisioned very differently.

One father who was unusually cool-headed stated, "I went in with an open mind, no definite ideas. So, actually, nothing unexpected happened and I remained calm."

Most labor coaches would find this emotional objectivity difficult to achieve. When labor hits a snag, fathers often wrestle with a common question: did some flaw in their coaching tip the balance?

"If I had been more effective, might the drugs have been avoided?" fretted one man after his wife was given medication to modify pain, which also resulted in her being too groggy to work effectively with her labor. Forceps-assisted births and cesareans are common medical interventions that trigger the same soul searching.

The answer is, probably not. So many factors influence the course of labor that something a coach does or does not do is unlikely to be able to change it significantly. Just the same, in his position as helper, a man usually feels a tremendous responsibility, especially when, as happened to Craig, the doctor or midwife considers his input in making a medical decision.

"Agreeing to medication that would strengthen contractions was a hard decision. I had no more of an idea what my wife was in for than she did, and the staff would only say that every woman's reaction was individual. Although the decision was clinched with the advice of the doctor and nurses, I felt in a way like I was throwing her to the wolves."

In Simon's case, the doctor respected his wish to delay a suggested change in labor management. Although the unborn baby seemed the right size to fit easily through his wife's pelvis, this normal downward movement was slow and his wife was growing tired.

"Our doctor was willing to go along with our request to wait a little longer before going ahead with the forceps. My wife was really trying and I didn't want her to feel she hadn't had the best shot."

Seth and his wife—whose fifth pregnancy was the first that didn't end in miscarriage—had hoped ardently for an uncomplicated birth. But he became one of the fathers who initiated intervention.

"We had a cesarean after twenty-four hours of hard labor. I began to feel desperate. I said to the doctor, 'We've got to do something. It's day and it's night and it's day, and the labor is still going on.' It was like a scene from M*A*S*H. We came to the decision that it had to end."

Fathers going through retrospective agonies of guilt and self-doubt might be heartened by Seth's philosophy:

"What are your alternatives after a certain point? You can always say, 'What if. . . ? Could I have. . . ?' but that gets you nowhere. You have to believe in the decision you made as right for the time."

Men can be further reassured by remembering that the midwife and, ultimately, the doctor, always have the last word on medical intervention. They may seriously consider the wishes of a laboring couple, but theirs will be the final decision based on professional knowledge and experience.

More and more men who are present for labor stay on for all medical procedures, including cesarean births. They agree that understanding procedures goes a long way toward eliminating qualms. More and more, men tend to ask "why" and "how" instead of following medical directives unquestioningly. Unfortunately, a busy staff may not have time to pass along all the information a father needs to reassure him. Ironically, he may be slower to absorb what he hears, due to anxiety over the unexpected turn of events. Communication also breaks down when doctors and nurses are uneasy about the presence of a father.

Yet a husband can be an asset during a procedure. For a woman to lose her partner, the person she knows and trusts, just as labor has taken a critical turn, is devastating. Hank stressed that the bond between prospective parents should not be underestimated.

> "She needed me as much—no, more—in the operating room. She was calmer, having me there. Having a cesarean frightened me, too. I wanted to be with her to know what was happening. Being strong for her kept me strong for myself."

While Hank and Seth were not without qualms as they faced medical procedures, they were acclimated to the hospital atmosphere through hours in labor and pre-labor training.

> "I kept halfway hoping that the doctor would say I couldn't join in. I would have been very happy to stay outside, but he obviously took it for granted that I was coming. Now I'm glad I did. I watched every step from start to finish. It was like an assembly line. Everyone did the next step without being told as if they could do it in their sleep, so efficient, so precise. There was no question in my mind about her safety."

"Once the staff realized that I was going to stay put and not stroll around as if I were at a sideshow, they relaxed and became quite friendly and instructive. I think, frankly, it's a bit of a territorial thing. They don't like outsiders on their turf."

Sharing the experience, parents usually are better able to withstand disappointment, even tragedy. One father, whose child was born too early to survive, said, "Our sorrow was shared. We cried together then and grieved together in the days afterward. We could understand and support each other because we had gone through our loss together."

Women often feel responsible for physical limitations that steer their labors onto unexpected courses. They reproach themselves and worry that they have disappointed their husbands. In fact, men are more likely to be compassionate than critical under these circumstances. Their disappointment centers on the loss of a mutual dream, not an unsatisfactory performance. One father expressed what many feel when he stated that "we had been warned in class against expecting pipe-dream-perfect labors but it was still hard not to feel it had been for nothing. We had worked so hard for so many hours."

Hank recalled, "When I realized that there wasn't going to be that glorious delivery room scene, my morale fell. This went away when I redirected my thoughts to the baby's welfare and my wife's."

Seth added, "The scheduling of a cesarean gave the remainder of labor a time limit. I was relieved that she would suffer less." Like most men, Hank's and Seth's predominant concern was for their wives and babies.

Some fathers, like these, are surprised and happy to find that a birth that takes place under vastly different circumstances than they had in mind can still be joyous and enriching.

"Despite the last-minute necessity for oxygen and spinal anesthesia, my wife was alert and aware during the delivery and the moment of birth thrilled me more than I had ever anticipated."

"Because the baby was in trouble and needed to be born quickly, my wife received a general anesthesia and forceps were used. This meant I couldn't be present for the birth. The one compensating factor was that I got to hold the baby almost immediately because my wife was in recovery. I bonded with him first, for a whole hour. I was unbelievably moved. And I could fill her in on his appearance when I saw her."

Because such grand scale medical intervention is usually sudden, questions and personal emotions arise after the fact. Seth needed to examine what happened in order to resolve doubts, anger, disappointment, and sorrow that took him by surprise after the cesarean was over.

"I needed to talk with other people and get it straight in my mind that what happened had to happen. My wife's parents were good about asking questions and I was grateful for the opportunity of working it through."

Everything that happens during labor should be seen as part of a whole. Both parents must value their efforts, not as performances that failed to match expectations, but as praiseworthy, even heroic accomplishments. The sense of union that a man and woman gain from working together so closely can be highly rewarding.

Finally, wondrously, there is the baby. Said Hank:

"Well, it's still our baby's birth, isn't it! That's what it's all about. I can't say I don't regret winding up with a Cecil B. DeMille production, but I look at the pluses. Certainly our hanging in there together is one. And getting this crazy, wonderful kid is another."

6 Birth and After

For most women, labor moves along without major detours. Once the opening to the uterus has stretched wide enough to slip over the baby's head, the birthing begins. Eric remembers:

"When the doctor announced that the baby would arrive soon, I was ecstatic. My wife was transformed, after seeming close to exhaustion. The prospect of victory after so many hours was a real high."

Now the infant is pushed from the uterus downward through the vagina, a marvelously elastic passageway whose muscular walls slowly unfold to let the baby pass. Officially, this is called the second stage of labor.

For a first-time mother, the second stage lasts an average of two hours; for other mothers, much less. Pressure from the baby's head on the mother's pelvic floor tissues stimulates an irresistible, tremendously forceful urge to push or bear down. This sensation, fleetingly comparable to the force behind a bowel movement, feels more like the mighty effort it would take to urge a giant boulder into motion single-handed. "She roared at the top of her lungs with each push," Simon remembered. "I was electrified by the power expressed in that sound."

Contraction by contraction, the baby descends, slipping back slightly after each push is over, moving forward again with the next one. Birth is real now, close at hand. The staff cheers the mother on while her husband physically supports her as she works.

"Our bodies were in contact as she pushed, I holding her from behind," recalled Andre. "The sensation for me was of us both giving birth. Exhilarating!"

There comes an incredible moment when a small, wet section of the baby's scalp appears at the mother's vaginal opening, showing larger and larger with each push. Eric remembered:

> "Seeing the baby's hair made it real that there was a person in there after all. I got so excited I jumped up on the bed. I was pushing as hard as she was."

With the birth imminent, the mother may be moved to the delivery room, as Craig's wife was. If she is in a less traditional setting, she is more likely to remain where she is, delivering in bed or in a birthing chair.

> "In the labor room, my reality was her pain. But when they rolled her into that delivery room, and I knew it really was going to happen, it seemed like, in that short period of time, the whole world stopped turning, and we were the center of it."

This is the moment that both mother and father have waited for ever since the pregnancy was confirmed: the birth of their child. After an unpredictable number of long, powerful pushes, all at once there is a splash of water from the uterus, some blood, and the infant slides from the mother's body. Eric and Clarence recalled their reactions:

> "As the baby sloshed out, the midwife caught him, swooped up his fat, pink body, and placed him in my wife's arms, all in one movement. Except for some

gurgling and clearing of his nasal passages, he lay quietly, his eyes open. We hung on to him tightly, he was so wet and slippery. I have never known a moment of such serenity. I was speechless."

"She seemed to fly out into the world, howling and wriggling all over, not at all the smiling infant in Leboyer's book. In my work I'm used to watching things develop step by step, bit by bit. Yet here was a whole person. I was seeing stars. She cried and cried, and I laughed aloud."

For many fathers, the physicality of birth is the moment of truth. Now, worries about becoming nauseated or faint may be realized. Experience shows that most men—like Craig and Pat—transcend this preoccupation.

"I had been worried about fainting at the sight of blood. But when the time came I watched the entire birth, including the episiotomy, and nothing fazed me at all. I checked out everything. My eyes were glued to that scene. I was in rapture watching."

"I was flying on one wing and a prayer, but it wasn't working. When I saw the baby I really started spinning, and I said aloud to no one in particular, 'I'm going to pass out.' Two nurses came over and put my head down between my legs and some smelling salts under my nose. In a few minutes I felt fine. They were so matter-of-fact that I wasn't even embarrassed."

A man's inhibitions may dissolve, moved as he is by seeing his child born. Love, tenderness, joy, relief, even a temporary numbness are among the many reactions men have to childbirth. Every response is individual, unpredictable, non-programmable, and beyond judgment. Simon couldn't stop his tears. "After all that work, all that waiting, wondering if they would use the forceps, the relief was tremendous. For once, I had no thought of self-consciousness, just letting the tears come."

Pat admitted that his primary feeling was of relief that it was over and everyone was safe. He said, "Mostly I was detached, a little ashamed that I wasn't measuring up, disappointed not to be experiencing the high the other fathers described. Later I realized how labor had shaken me. I was in beyond my depth and I suppose I needed some space until I had absorbed it all."

Birth brings the future closer, bridging time, putting some men in touch with their own mortality. Through their children, Nicholas and Simon saw the continuance of themselves.

> "As I first saw her, looking like a sleepy little gnome who had just been pulled out from behind a tree stump, the profoundness of my feelings astonished me. I thought, with jubilation and pride, 'This is *my* child, my flesh and blood.'"

> "Old age had always seemed eons away. In this instant the concept of a lifetime shrank to something suddenly measurable. I saw my child as representing a new generation, which moved me ahead to another time. Old age no longer seemed so far ahead as to be unimaginable."

The first direct encounter with his child is an unforgettable moment for every father. Their relationship starts with this first meeting. Andre described the moment:

"She lay there like a delicate rosy flower, softly breathing. I felt my heart open to her and take her in. I will probably live the rest of my life without experiencing such unguarded joy and relief."

"She didn't come out so pretty and that startled me, putting me off a little bit," Pat recalled. "I said so and the doctor said, 'Don't start judging her now,' and that was some of the greatest advice I ever got. All I can say is she has certainly shaped up since."

Jordan summed up this special experience: "I knew that our relationship would be forever special because I was right there seeing my child from time zero. It's such an important experience. There is no way to replace it. I can't imagine all those generations of men who didn't have it for their own. What would that be like? The father is outside and all of a sudden hears this baby. He has no idea how it all happened, how his baby came into being part of this world."

Fathers like Scott and Charlie who have been absent from the labor and birth and are introduced to a *fait accompli* already bundled in a blanket are more likely to feel disconnected and ambivalent toward their babies.

"The nurse brought the baby to me in the waiting room, swaddled in blankets with only a red, puckered face showing. I could not take in that this was the child— *my* child—that my wife had carried inside her for nine months."

"I had no attachment to him after he was born. I didn't know who this baby, this new person, was. He was simply there in a crib in the nursery. How could I have feelings for him? They said, 'This is your son,' but it was weeks before I had any connection with him."

A father may feel even more detached if he had to wait out a cesarean birth, as Kevin wound up doing. Fortunately, alienation is not inevitable for men who do not attend their babies' births. Kevin had an urgent desire to greet his child at the earliest possible opportunity. "I wouldn't put up with seeing my baby through a nursery window. I just wanted to hold him really badly and demanded that I be allowed to do it."

Studies show that most new fathers, including those not present for the birth, who at least hold their babies, share eye contact and in some way care for them very soon afterward, generally feel close to their children early on. Early attachment appears to carry over into the home, with fathers more inclined to spend time voluntarily with their newborns and to care for them earlier and more often than fathers who missed this opportunity. Certainly, when the nurses brought Kevin's baby to him, his reaction spoke for itself: "He was given to me to hold. At that moment his eyes opened and we looked at each other. Never before have I felt such a powerful connection with any person as I did at that moment."

Eric was equally moved. "I had briefly and very awkwardly held one infant before. But when I held *my* baby it was like I had done it all my life."

In the final analysis, according to fathers who have participated in labor and birth, something extra special happens between them and their babies only in the presence of the birth itself. Men who have shared this experience with their wives and babies stress its importance for them as fathers. Hank and Clarence exulted:

"If I'd waited in the waiting room, as I'd originally thought I preferred, I would have been pleased and proud. But the nurses wouldn't have had to keep pulling me down off the ceiling. That's the key. I don't know if it's adrenalin, but something hit me and it wasn't just a sheer cerebral thing. I can't imagine that I would have the relationship that I have with my son now if I had just been presented with a kid wrapped in a bundle."

"It's a result of experiencing the birth that the level of joy is so extreme. I wouldn't think of giving out stinking old cigars because they are so mundane. It's the process— going through the pain, trying, failing, succeeding, watching the birth, whatever you do—that peaks with the arrival of the baby. You don't get that if you're not there. It's the emotional bridge that takes you into the greater potential."

Afterward

In most birthing centers and a few hospitals, father, mother, and the newly born baby remain united until they all leave for home together. Usually they can depart within a few hours following birth, if mother and child are in stable condition.

More often, in hospitals, after a short time together the new family is separated. The baby is taken to the nursery for a period of observation, the mother to her room to rest, and the father disengages from the rarified atmosphere of which he has been a part and re-enters the ordinary, everyday world.

How does a man feel, a new father on his own with the drama of labor and birth now behind him? Hank, having witnessed one of life's greatest miracles, no longer saw himself as the same person.

"Having been present for the birth changed my life. It opened up a realm of consciousness I never had before. I felt expanded as a human being, newly inspired about life's possibilities. LSD is small potatoes in comparison."

Looking back, Andre said, "I was glad to be home alone because there I could get really silly about it, jumping up and down, screaming, hooting and hollering. I was elated for days."

But beyond this celebrating there is another level of feelings. When a new father reports to relatives and friends, he seldom refers to the hard work or the emotional pain he has experienced. He may not even think of them. Birth, the climax to nine months of anticipation capped by hours of concentrated effort, sweeps aside the memory of stress. Once he is alone and quiet, however, no longer insulated by challenge and excitement, he is vulnerable to the emotional aftermath of all he has gone through. These fathers describe their reactions:

"Birth was a positive memory, but very intense. The smell of the amniotic fluid was strong in my mind for a long time. It made me realize how little I knew about how I felt about birth. I was shocked to realize I didn't know."

"I was relieved the pregnancy was over. The strain of it all had been more than I realized. As for the birth, I

wouldn't have missed that for anything. But mostly I
felt numb because of my physical and mental exhaustion and my reaction to everything that had gone on in
labor. I walked around pretty spaced out until my wife
got home. I had trouble speaking to people. They
would call and it was like, 'Yeah. . .talk to you in a
couple of days.'"

"Once I got home, it hit me like a ton of bricks. I cried
myself to sleep. The next day, when anyone called and
said, 'How did it go?' I burst into tears. When my wife
phoned, sounding just like any other day, and asked
how I was doing, I burst into tears again and had to
hang up and call her back. It was almost as though I
was going through my own personal pain for what she
experienced the day before."

A man's distress over seeing the woman he loves in
pain and his relative helplessness to stop it often lingers for
a long time. Reconciliation to this part of his experience
seems to be difficult, particularly as the age-old question of
how to relieve the pain of labor without jeopardizing mother
or baby remains inadequately answered to this day. He may
more readily come to terms with disappointment over his
performance as coach. Initially, as he looks back over labor
and birth, he tends to judge his helpfulness by what he
observed—the degree to which his wife was in control of
her relaxation and breathing, how effectively she stayed on
top of pain. At times, the experience is totally rewarding for
both parents, as it was for Jordan.

More commonly, men find themselves both frustrated
and rewarded, depleted and enriched by their experience.
Too often, it is what didn't work that sways self-assessment.
Despite a commendable track record, especially considering

how difficult labor was, Seth jumped to the conclusion that he had failed as a coach.

> "Sharing labor was beautiful and I felt I'd been pretty helpful, but I'm the kind of person who always thinks I could have done better, tried harder. The coaching was more difficult than classes had led me to believe. Whatever I tried appeared to have so little effect compared with what I wanted for her. The breathing being less effective than I expected was the biggest disappointment. We worked as hard as we could just to keep her from going to pieces, and sometimes we couldn't even achieve that. It was an endless, exhausting endurance test. At the end I was thrilled—but I still felt I had let her down and was discouraged about that."

Seth's self-condemnation was probably unwarranted. This is true for a majority of coaches. Most women, too preoccupied to offer feedback to their husbands during labor, later say, "I couldn't have made it without him." These new mothers speak movingly of their feelings:

> "I think my husband was most important to me from an emotional standpoint. Without his love and encouragement, I couldn't have made it."

> "I did not by any means experience a painless childbirth, but my husband's presence there beside me was such a comfort."

> "Every time I thought I couldn't handle it any longer, seeing my husband's strong face and hearing his voice got me back on the track."

"The joy of being together for the birth of our son was most precious of all to me."

In reflecting on labor as a whole, both parents can confuse disappointment with failure. Every couple starts by hoping for the perfect birth, which colors expectations. A man who concludes that he has failed because his actual experiences differed from those he expected, ranging anywhere from a cesarean instead of a vaginal birth to the failure of breathing to produce painless contractions, throws away much that is valuable.

Feelings of disappointment, anger, sorrow, frustration are real and must be acknowledged. But it is also important for a man to value what he did do rather than what he couldn't do, as Hank pointed out:

"The labor was long and horrendous, and I was not as patient as I would like to have been. It's easy to knock yourself over the head in retrospect. But I'm not going to have myself shot at dawn for the things I couldn't help. I did my best, and that's cause for celebration right there."

For a man to see himself as a failure when he has just achieved the supreme status of fatherhood is a tragic self-limitation. The bond formed by teamwork and sharing the arrival of a child, whatever the circumstances, cannot be underestimated.

Another very positive outcome for many couples is a man's increased admiration and respect for his wife after he sees her through childbirth. The special endurance and vigor that are inherent in women and that often surface for the first time during labor and birth deeply impress all who observe it. Jordan was profoundly moved.

"After seeing her give birth, I can only say that I respect how strong my woman is, and how positive, and how strong all mothers must be to go through this and then taking care of a child. My image of my mate and of women couldn't be higher."

Andre summed up his experience: "Working so intensely together brought us closer. Each of us put everything we've got into it. It's one more irreplaceable experience you have together that further solidifies your relationship."

Now three people face a future together—two adults and one small baby. A new adventure is underway: the beginning of learning in many ways, a continuation of growth and change.

POSTBIRTH

"Having a child takes you out of yourself and at the same time focuses you directly in on yourself, and in so doing, centers you. It takes you into the universe and your place there."

7 Feeling Like a Father

On the day following his son's birth, the new father opens his front door and steps out into the sunshine. Exalted by his new status, he looks about him. Surely the air is fresher, the sky more blue. Even the puppy tearing up his newspaper is sort of cute. He glances at the headlines. Glum as ever. His neighbor appears, nods—"Hear you had a boy! Congratulations!"—and hurries off to work. A few blocks away, rush hour is in full force. The new father frowns:

> "Realizing that the topsy-turvy state of the world hadn't gone away, I felt, 'Don't you understand? The world's changed. I'm a *father!*' But the earth didn't stop turning because I had a baby. What a let-down!"

He reminds himself that, at work, where he is known, things will be different. He strides into the office, beaming, his good spirits restored. But he is in for a disappointing surprise.

> "Back on the job I heard, 'Congratulations! Now, about this order . . . ' I was half-way through the first day before I stopped resenting the casualness."

The new father is puzzled, embarrassed, maybe even a little bitter. Certainly he feels different. Not unreasonably, he expects others to acknowledge the change. Instead, he receives the impression that, in the eyes of the world around him, fatherhood rates a fairly ordinary response.

Such scenarios are not unfamiliar to many new fathers. It may be at moments like these, after the cheers and congratulations have died down, that the man who walked out of the delivery room with his own exalted visions of fatherhood begins to realize that he is not so sure after all what being a father means, beyond the time-honored commitment to feed, clothe, and protect his child.

In recent years, fathers have been changing their expectations and behavior, yet their image remains close to what it once was. Traditional attitudes stick like old-fashioned glue. Despite fathers' involvement in pregnancy, their presence at birth, and their increased share in baby care, the society in which they live continues to see their participation as secondary, rather than as an expression of their equal importance in producing a child.

For example, while many hospitals have expanded visiting privileges to admit fathers throughout the day and evening, fathers and babies can be together for only an hour or so every three to four hours when the newborns leave the nursery for scheduled feedings, unless mother and baby share a room round the clock. Said Hank, "I had expected more than the chance to hold my son briefly after he'd finished nursing or a quick diaper change before the nurse whisked him away."

Absence from work can be another problem. A man's boss is inclined to be less sympathetic in granting him time off to be with his new family than to attend services for the death of a relative, for example, or a religious holiday. Setting aside vacation time in advance is always a possibility, but most often due dates are not perfectly predictable. Money and position are top priorities in a man's world, and most businesses look at a man in terms of his career, not in terms of his family. Time off for a new baby is viewed as a favor, not a right.

The comments of these three fathers typify what many new fathers say about spending time with their new families soon after birth:

"I took as much time as I could, but when I went back to work I wanted to be with them. I missed them so, I used to go home at lunch time."

"I didn't like going off to work and leaving my daughter behind. I'd already had my vacation, so it would have meant no salary if I took time off."

"I didn't want to ask for too much time off. It would have looked like I didn't take my job seriously."

Relatives, too, often see a father differently than he sees himself. Charlie told of heated arguments with his in-laws over whether they or he should drive mother and baby home from the hospital. He insisted, but they showed up on departure day for a final wrangle in the parking lot. Several men described power struggles with their wives' mothers or even their own, over how best to help out at home. In these instances, fathers were credited with only secondary status, their ideas and efforts dismissed.

Eric found that even physicians can have this attitude.

"Our pediatrician asked me to have my *wife* call if there were further questions during one illness. Needless to say, I made sure *I* called. I let him know that, as a father, I had as much concern with my child's health as her mother did, and he had better learn to deal with fathers."

Finally, fathers themselves are divided when it comes to the degree and quality of their involvement with the baby. Pat felt alienated and defensive around several of his buddies, whose companionship he usually enjoyed, when he realized how their attitudes differed from his.

> "Cigars with little pink or blue bands, a clap on the back, watching football games while mom changes the wet diaper—that's what they were into. I was like a piece of putty around my daughter at home, cooed and made faces at her along with my wife. I even changed diapers. But Saturday afternoons when we all got together I felt a little foolish and backed off. I didn't like playing down how much I cared."

How have we arrived at this playing down of the emotional importance of fatherhood, at seeing men's involvement with their children as less important than women's? Traditional images of fathering, handed down over time, show us fathers who are aloof from household affairs, removed from the frustrations and rewards of caring for children by their involvement with earning a living in the outside world. Only mothers are expected to hover, worry, and melt with love, to be emotionally involved with assimilating a child into their lives. Fathers, historically and currently, frequently are presented either as fleeing from responsibility, looking on with awe, or—presto!—confidently absorbed into family life. Their emotional transition from being childless to being fathers is largely unexplored. Father images in television, film, and advertising bring dad into the kitchen but wind up being too romantically superficial to apply to real life. Often a television father is portrayed as competent and nurturing only when the mother is permanently absent.

Generally speaking, fathers continue to be seen as basically self-sufficient, worldly, objective, reserved, mind-centered—characteristics suitable for their position as head of the family. Mothers, who retain their monopoly as the nurturers of infants and children, are expected to be soft, intuitive, receptive, heart-centered.

Today's men want very much to be more loving and sensitive in relationships. For a father who is deeply touched when he holds his newborn child, the potential for nurturing is obvious. Yet desire alone is not enough to break with tradition.

Many men say they are disconcerted to realize that they are not at all certain how to take the step from *becoming* a father to *feeling like* a father. After spending time at home with his baby son, Hank, who had been ecstatic when he was born, had to admit, "A piece was missing. It felt unreal, like I was an imposter. That was disturbing because I didn't know where it was supposed to come from. I expected to be flooded with some newfound maturity, reliability. But I felt none of that."

Here is a man filled with excitement over having a child, but feeling lost because he has not, as yet, grasped a more complete sense of emotional involvement as a father. This aspect of his role is so alien that he feels, to quote another father, "like an imposter." Many men see fatherhood as conflicting in part with the identity they already know—their own. "What I was looking for," Hank explained, "was how I, as an individual, fit into being a father without losing track of myself."

Until the two identities meshed, a trade-off seemed necessary to him, a giving up of his personal identity for certain ways of thinking and behaving that he saw as appropriate to being a father. Other fathers had similar reactions:

"As I considered my role as a father versus other men's roles as fathers, I felt like I was supposed to outfit myself with a pipe and slippers or something. That simply wasn't me."

"When you have a family, people see you differently. I don't want the only reason that I exist to be because I am a father. To be expected to respond like a father makes me feel like I am walking on eggshells. I can relate best to people as *me*, who also happens to be a father."

"At first I was still myself versus fatherhood. One hadn't yet blended with the other. This seemed to be something that I would allow to happen when I was certain that I would still remain a separate person, an individual. At first I wasn't quite sure I still existed as myself—like, wait a minute, I can still do things on my own."

New fathers want to be involved—but they do not want to be swallowed up by a classic character part arbitrarily assigned to fathers. Sometimes, the pull to be emotionally connected contrasts with feelings that urge retreat, as Seth discovered during his early weeks as a father.

"I found myself taking a longer route to come home from work, adding twenty minutes to an already lengthy drive. Then I'd find myself driving down the street where we lived before my son was born. I caught myself saying, 'This is so symbolic, I can't stand it!'"

The powerful, unfamiliar emotions triggered by becoming a father may also cause a man to back off from his new

role. "Nothing ever made me feel different until this baby,"
explained Simon. "All the feelings I had before were
knowns, just experienced to a greater or lesser degree."

Fathers say that, while the passionate responses elicited
by the birth and presence of a child may be startling, they
are not necessarily unwelcome, just new. When a new father feels overwhelmed as he searches for his own niche, he
may temporarily distance himself to get his bearings. Ironically, some fathers, like Kevin, find their jobs—where fatherhood is played down—to be reassuring.

> "It was a relief to get back into the swing of my usual
> life. Leaving home for work, I thought, 'Yes, it's still
> here. I'm still here.' It was important for me to get back
> to work, to re-establish my familiar life."

Traditional prescriptions for fatherhood are too limiting
to suit our changing times. The only emotional parenting
image a father usually has to go by is that of "mother." But
the nurturing feelings expressed by fathers are not simply
mothers' feelings transferred. They are feelings that reflect
male attitudes and viewpoints. Men are not looking to take
on mothering roles but to respond as fathers, as men, as
themselves.

In fact, the time-honored roles of protector, provider,
link with the world, can serve as starting points. These fathers expressed that viewpoint:

> "As I stood looking at this tiny sleeping child, I was
> struck by his total helplessness and overwhelmed by
> anxiety lest I prove inadequate to take proper care of
> him. This was my child, totally dependent on me to
> keep him from harm."

"Now I have to be serious at home, to be totally there as a real person. This is the one thing in my life that is going to last forever. It is up to me to keep this together. The feeling isn't heavy but a good feeling, natural and right. We have an investment here, something I see happening every day in front of my eyes, a momentous thing."

"You know how you believe certain things but they get washed out of everyday life. Then something happens to focus you back on it and strengthen it for you. All of a sudden I have a child, and I want her to know that I have a sense of value about myself so that she will have a sense of value about herself, too."

Men agree that the fuller sense of fatherhood comes only through living with their babies. Feeling like a father takes root slowly. It is a product of time and experience blended with individual personality and goals, an understanding that comes only retrospectively. As Hank discovered:

"There was never one particular stunning moment of realization. I took in the idea of myself as a father gradually. Fatherhood is like birth. You can anticipate it, but there's nothing like experiencing it."

That experience starts the day a newborn baby arrives at home.

8 Baby Care

When Seth brought his wife and baby home from the hospital, he was nervous and uncertain. Having joyfully anticipated being an important part of his baby's life, he had become disconcerted by his reaction to his son after spending only a few hours each evening with him in the hospital.

"The baby was really a stranger. This was our child, but who was it? Someone we like? Friend or foe? It was unsettling for us both. We had been expecting someone and no one, including the baby, knew the outcome. Once he arrived, this stranger, we had an eerie feeling because now this someone was real, a little person doing things."

Seth's lack of connection with his child, his perception that this incredibly small and fragile being was as alien as a visitor from Mars, was intensified by the way his son looked and behaved. Indeed, to uninitiated parents, even those who dote on their infants, newborns can seem pretty peculiar.

Their skins, wrinkled and peeling, and often yellow or red in color instead of pink, can be dotted with rashes and tiny pimples. Newly born babies often have temporarily lopsided heads, crossed eyes, flat little noses, receding chins that quiver when they cry, bulging tummies, and bow legs. They grimace and twitch, breathe in irregular rhythms, and fling their arms wide in shaky responses when they are startled—evidence of nervous systems still under development.

Seth fully expected to help care for his baby, not simply pitching in to give his wife a break but in his own right as a father. But, like many fathers, he arrived home with a three-day-old baby just coming out of postbirth sleepiness, to whom he had barely been introduced. Having focused almost exclusively on the particulars of pregnancy and birth during recent months, he now realized that what he didn't know about baby care suddenly seemed immeasurable. Doing everything right struck him as crucial. "I was afraid of looking incompetent," he explained. "I was embarrassed that other fathers would do better, that I'd be shown up."

Because men tend to compete with each other for competency, they usually keep self-doubt to themselves. Rather than expose their uncertainties, new fathers are likely to exchange questions and answers briefly and seemingly casually. So Seth, like many new fathers, had no way of knowing that his worries were very common. And when he tentatively sought feedback from his acquaintances, he found their generalized comments like, "Play it by ear," and "Do whatever comes naturally," meaningful only in retrospect.

Seth was entering a new role for which he had no precedent. It is not just the baby, the attendant responsibility, and the lack of skills that are alien to a new father. The whole situation is a mystery, especially for men who, in electing to become more involved parents than the generations of fathers before them—or even many of their contemporaries—have thrown off traditional guidelines and entered the uncharted territory of baby care. For Seth, the result was chaos.

"The first days were like a Keystone Cops comedy with both of us running around wondering how to handle everything. There were the two of us, four hands, changing a diaper, needing a third person to fetch things, to tell us what to do. I wanted basic one, two, three steps, but it doesn't work out that way. Things form their own rhythm. Eventually you realize it's not an emergency every time something happens. But until then, the old jokes don't play too well."

Baby care, like any skill, is learned. For years, mothers have been cast as baby care mavins, creating the popular but false impression that women, not men, have special talents for burping and bathing babies. One father, who observed, "Looking at my wife with the baby I was amazed. She was a natural," wouldn't have argued with this view. But the truth is that mothers, just like fathers, start as novices.

Craig's wife was a nurse, but the extra measure of security that gave him when he left the hospital with his new family was short-lived. "In fact," he recalled, "she was very nervous and I ended up being more supportive of her. She felt that, as a mother, she *should* know, *couldn't* fall apart, *had* to be cool."

"I expected my wife to know how to take care of the baby because she was the mother," said Nicholas. "She expected me to know because I work with little children in my job. It was just as crazy for me to think that she knew everything because she is a woman, as it was for her to expect that I should know because I studied developmental psychology."

Sigmund Freud formalized the myth that women are especially talented in caring for babies. He believed that men do not have the sensitive, softly affectionate responses to babies that he assumed were instinctive to women. When he observed that fathers held themselves aloof from their children and that mothers were the involved nurturing parents, Freud neglected to consider the influence of the Victorian environment of his time. Only recently have his conclusions been disputed as fact.

In fact, gentle, tender feelings toward babies are very definitely present in both sexes. Although hormones released when a woman gives birth probably play a part in triggering this response for her, environment and circumstances can set it off or stifle it for either parent. Recent research shows that men become deeply absorbed with their newborns when they can see and touch them early on, even when they have sized themselves up as the detached type of father. Parental attitudes, like skills, are learned.

Clarence was representative of many of today's fathers who, having inherited the mythical legacy that men are insensitive to babies, are challenging it. Intent on following their hearts instead of censoring them, they are establishing a new tradition: fathers' nurturing involvement in baby care. The drawback is that they have few guidelines.

Women, Clarence's wife included, often approach baby care backed by an immense amount of information, gleaned largely from books. But Clarence himself, along with most of the men whose experiences are reflected in this book, did little or no reading. When asked why, fathers often replied, "Too busy," or "She does the reading for both of us." Why, really, did they not read? Was it a way of avoiding an unknown that was too frightening to look at directly? Would it have been an admission of ignorance and, thus, inadequacy? A crossing of forbidden or intimidating boundaries into women's territory?

On one level, the stereotype of being seen as peripheral to baby care may work as an advantage for men. Because mothers customarily are in charge of early parenting, some new fathers look to their wives for direction, feeling safer, as they learn, with things in "expert hands."

"She became the boss, in charge of everything," Hank explained, obviously relieved. "This was contrary to our usual relationship. Normally I'm considered the rock. In this case I relied on her to know what to do. After all, she was the mother."

But Hank's reliance on his wife as the expert caused friction when she couldn't answer all his questions. "We had some battles over this," he recalled. "She'd say, 'Well, why are you asking *me*?' Then, when she didn't come through, I got mad."

Seth, who approached fathering differently, feeling his way along, cautiously coming up with a suggestion now and then, found that he became nervous when his wife agreed with his ideas. "All of a sudden I was in charge," he said. "She had given up her control for a moment."

Perhaps the information in books was not what men needed to know about caring for babies? Clarence offered an explanation:

"I don't believe that knowing how to put on a diaper would have changed how I felt. Or how to hold a bottle. Or the twelve and a half steps of giving a bath. You're in awe of this little thing. It's like dynamite in a small package. Handle with care!"

The subject of how to respond emotionally to new babies tends to get left out of formal instruction on baby care. Perhaps that invisible, heart-centered aspect of parenting is what Clarence was trying to express.

"My wife read so much that I was concerned she would do it by the book, rigidly, not spontaneously. I really wanted to learn—but as an overall, not getting into the mechanics of it. I wanted it to come from inside me, from my kid, from *us*, not from books."

The vision of women as authorities on baby care may release some men from the pressure to come up with all the answers. Relatively unencumbered, they may feel free to be spontaneous. Seth concluded, "I wanted to be taught, and yet I didn't. It's like getting a new car and being the first one to drive it. I didn't want anything to cloud this brand-new experience."

When a Woman Breastfeeds

Breastfeeding is another aspect of baby care that proved to be both an asset and a liability in relationships with their wives, said several fathers.

"In my opinion, there is nothing more beautiful than the human connection between mother and child during breastfeeding," observed Craig, moved by his experience when his wife nursed their baby. Many fathers, Clarence and Andre among them, also react with pleasure and appreciation.

"For me it was a turn-on in the sense that it was another aspect of a woman being a woman, as feminine as she can be. I took a picture of my wife breastfeeding our one-day-old baby. Now, two years later, I still have it on the tie clip bar in my jewelry box because I still like to look at it."

"I thought breastfeeding was fascinating. What, for years, I'd seen only as a source of sexual pleasure I now realized also worked in a different way, like a piece of equipment. The dual function was exciting and interesting to me. I found my wife much more attractive. The potential of her breasts enhanced her femaleness."

On the flip side, there are men, like Kevin, who respond pragmatically rather than poetically.

> "We were both breastfed as babies, so it seemed perfectly natural. There's no question that it is healthiest for a new baby. For me it was no big deal, just perfectly logical."

Babies are nourished at their mothers' breasts the world over, although the custom all but disappeared in the United States when baby formula was introduced and bottle feeding became stylish. Breastfeeding came back into vogue in the 1960s close on the heels of interest in natural childbirth, as women attempted to personalize birthing and the events that surround it. More and more parents now understand that human milk, especially geared to human babies, is easiest to digest, naturally laxative, germ-free and rich with antibodies appropriate for growing infants. However, with formula manufacturing companies campaigning diligently to keep up sales, nearly half the babies in the United States are still given formula. Charlie's comment reflects the dichotomy that continues regarding breastfeeding versus bottle feeding:

> "I would have been happier with bottles and formula like everybody else we knew. Why go out of your way to be different? Breastfeeding was for our grandmothers."

Our society's runaway sex consciousness still categorizes breasts mainly as sexual objects. Instead of feeling admiration or even nonchalance at the sight of a mother nursing her baby, some people are ill at ease, occasionally vehemently opposed. This was Eric's experience with relatives at a Thanksgiving reunion:

"I was surprised to see my brother-in-law walk out of the room in embarrassment when my wife opened her blouse to nurse. It seemed pretty silly because you can see more when she's in her bathing suit. He never objected to that."

Other fathers described their experiences:

"In the park, an enraged woman marched up to my wife and said that nursing in public was indecent exposure, corrupting her two sons playing nearby."

"I felt very awkward among strangers. It's just not common here and even though my wife was discreet, we always got lots of curious, sometimes hostile stares. I think many people really do regard it as a peep show."

Some fathers, like the following, see breastfeeding as highly personal, more suited to a private setting. Reasons need not be puritanical.

"I found myself protective of her wish not to breastfeed in public even though I was perfectly comfortable with it. In fact, originally I tried to get her to feel more at ease with it. Ultimately, I felt it most important that she be able to relax and feel good about what she was doing."

"It seemed to us an intimate part of our new life as a family that we preferred to keep for ourselves alone. There's always a spot that you can have for yourselves for the hour or so a feeding takes."

These men recognized an element that is absolutely essential for breastfeeding to succeed: the absence of emotional and physical tension. Feeling positive about the act of nursing enables a woman to relax physically during feedings, thus permitting her milk to flow freely. Babies, keenly perceptive, tune in to the emotions of the person feeding them, accepting the feeding most readily when they, too, are calm and relaxed.

To the uninitiated, nursing looks easy: no expense, nothing to prepare, no waste, no garbage. But there is more than meets the eye. Babies want to eat when they are hungry, not by timed schedules. Because breast milk is so easily digested, newborns tend to nurse every two hours at least. This puts a huge demand on a nursing mother's time and patience, even though she is enthusiastic and willing. Whether she succeeds at breastfeeding depends in part on her husband's attitude. She may be overwhelmed and give up if he, as the person who is with her most often, is disapproving, uninterested, ambivalent, or jealous. "Knowing where I stood made it easier for her to manage," said one man.

Pat was basically in favor of breastfeeding. But he saw the attention he once received being rerouted to his daughter. He was also concerned lest his baby become more attached to his wife than to him.

> "Mom and baby were getting a lot of satisfaction through nursing, establishing a loving closeness that used to be mine. This made me feel cut off more than anything else."

Scott, like many fathers, regretted the impossibility of nursing the baby himself. He mourned missing the singular, intimate relationship breastfeeding provides. He felt this most keenly when the baby cried and breastfeeding was the only way he could be consoled.

"I could hold the baby, amuse him, rock him to sleep, but I couldn't breastfeed him. Sometimes he quieted only with his mother. That's when I was helpless. Logically, I knew I couldn't nurse, but I still missed it. It's like there's a piece missing in me."

Some men, like Kevin, support breastfeeding as soundly practical but find that this new function of breasts diminishes their appeal.

"I was one hundred percent for it, and still am. The one drawback is that, since I've seen my wife's breasts in a different light, I don't find them as attractive as I did before."

Clarence reacted differently: "She was like a different woman. I was totally in love again. It wasn't overly important, but something new adds spice. And she felt more responsive, sexier, because I was more aware."
Lovemaking can be affected negatively when a father is unable to harmonize his reactions to the combined sexual and biological functions of his wife's breasts. Although Nicholas felt sometimes that he was "in bed with a milk factory," he concluded that:

"Being more playful helped me not to take everything so personally, like it was all coming down on me. I had a feeling of irony. The baby and I shared her breasts. We were each getting our nourishment in different ways. It was amusing, although adjusting to the baby's part in it was difficult at first."

When fathers can recognize their reservations and discuss them with their wives, solutions usually are possible.

Hank, for example, took a practical view of his wife's singular ability to calm their crying son: "I was relieved that she could take over and get him to be quiet. It was better than hearing him scream and it was a built-in break for me."

For most fathers, the solution lies in entering the breastfeeding experience in their own way. Pat put it like this:

> "I realized finally that it wasn't an exclusive duet they were doing. It's really that my wife wasn't appealing *directly* to me as she was during the pregnancy and before. To continue to be involved, *I* had to find a way."

Here is an opportunity for a father to adapt his traditional role as protector to current needs. By shielding his nursing wife in public—"I stood in front of her when she nursed," said one man—arranging private space to feed the baby, helping his wife to get the nutrition and rest she needs to produce plenty of milk, a father is standing up for his family in ways that no one else can.

Several men said they compensated by actively involving themselves at feeding time. Simon related:

> "I always got up with my wife at night when she breastfed because I enjoyed that private time together. It was the highlight of my day, a chance to talk when the baby was quietly with us."

Although some breastfeeding babies make it clear that, for them, only mother will do, others quite cheerfully switch occasionally to bottled breast milk. Scott had not known that this was a possibility.

"I hadn't even thought about it until my wife walked in one day with the bottle and said, 'Here! You feed him.' It was so much more meaningful than I thought it could be, holding my son in my arms while he was taking nourishment from me. It was definitely a peak moment."

Pat came up with another way to achieve a special closeness with his daughter, one that many fathers have discovered.

"I found that I could have some of that closeness by holding her against my bare chest when I relaxed in our hammock. This worked only after a feeding when she would lie quietly without nuzzling for the nipple. But it was lovely, one of the loveliest times we had together, totally peaceful, almost like we blended together."

Routine daily care, walks taken together, play, conversation, simple body contact—all are forms of communication that generate familiarity and intimacy.

Once babies are weaned, fathers who reminisce about the pros and cons of nursing tend to favor breastfeeding. Whatever their experiences—and most are mixed—top priority goes to the high quality of nourishment that breast milk gives babies during their early months. Pat summarized:

"In the end, I was glad we went that route. It was a great deal more practical—no mess, no expense—and the baby obviously has benefited, healthy and happy as she is."

Working Together as Partners

New fathers say they do not need to learn the how-tos of baby care as much as they need to learn self-reliance and confidence. One very real issue is the working-out of a baby-care partnership with their mates. Both men and women are perfectly capable of learning to care for babies. As people with differing personalities and values, each can contribute uniquely to their baby's care and development. Logically, one partner will prove to be more capable in certain areas than the other—depending, not on sex, but on personality and background.

"I feel more competent than my wife at certain things," said one man. "Bathing, for instance, seemed simpler to me, not as complex as she made it." His wife might have been delighted to turn over their baby's daily baths to him.

Another father observed, "It bothered me that she wasn't very affectionate with the baby." All women aren't gentle and loving, any more than all men are strong and silent.

"Right" or "wrong" is important only when the baby's comfort or health is at stake. Yet parents who are just starting to work toward a real partnership often get caught up in competing with each other. The comments of these two fathers show how this can happen.

"We had some fierce arguments over differences of opinion on our daughter's care. It felt like we were competing with each other for parent-of-the-month award."

"I was open to dressing our baby, giving it a whirl, but my wife was such a perfectionist that it was less of a hassle to bow out gracefully."

By retiring to the background, this father was sacrificing a certain level of involvement with his baby.

A new father should not have to hang back, bowing to the prevailing image of mothers as the "experts." Ideally, he will feel free to take over the care or cuddling he longs to give.

Ideally, parenting will be a partnership in which each parent respects the other's interest, ability, and right to be part of raising their child. Differences of opinion plus deep emotional investments are bound to trigger arguments, but as long as each parent can keep their mutual goals, rather than competition, in mind, these can be constructive exchanges.

Hank, whose relationship with his wife previously had fit the classic duo of wage-earner/homemaker, became a more understanding husband once he experienced firsthand the nitty-gritty of caring for a new baby.

"I used to come home at night to find supper not started, the bed still unmade, my wife in the same housecoat looking harassed. I was puzzled, wondering what she could possibly have been doing all day. When she got sick and went to her mother's for the weekend, and I wound up taking care of our son for three days, I understood. Even spending more than two minutes in the bathroom is a luxury. I had no concept of this before."

For Clarence, hands-on experience made a world of difference in the way he saw himself as an involved, nurturing father. He took such delight in caring for his baby that his original worries about competence were replaced with confidence and self-respect.

"When I dress my baby, I put on whatever is around. Not exactly a fashion show. In fact, my wife would change her ten minutes after I finished. Makes me feel annoyed in a small way, but I think it's kind of funny, too. *I* think she looks great. So what if the tags are in front. Someday, when she's in school, she'll still do okay. I see beyond the small stuff to the more important elements in life."

Developing a parenting partnership takes effort and time. Patience, self-esteem, and respect for each other's contributions, while invaluable assets, are not the only ingredients. Although it often is not immediately obvious, the baby plays a part, too—as we shall see in the next chapter.

9 Relating to a Newborn

Had they ever talked together, Hank and Clarence would have discovered that they had something very much in common. Like Seth, and many other new fathers, they could not seem to relate personally to their new babies—not only when they were a day or two old and peculiar-looking, but for several weeks after they were born. Tremendously moved by the birth of his child, filled with pride and a strong sense of protectiveness, each was secretly troubled by the feeling that, nevertheless, he and his child were strangers.

"For a couple of weeks I came home from work and forgot he was there," Seth said, laughing ruefully. "It would take a couple of minutes. I'd be walking around the house and then—'Oh!' " Normally tuned into his feelings, highly sensitive, he went on to say:

> "I realized this was my baby to take care of. I'd play with him, hold him, bathe him, all these things. Yet even though I involved myself physically from the start, I couldn't feel that special something toward him. This bothered me, and I felt responsible about not passing along any negative vibrations."

Hank, despite a fairly gloomy outlook about life with a baby, surprised himself. A distancer by nature, he was letting down his guard, and his son was the reason.

> "I figured it would be okay to have a baby around, but not great, probably a hindrance. There may be an

advantage to being a born pessimist. I expected everything to be horrible. It wasn't."

Nevertheless Hank found the invasion of his personal
life irritating. One reason: The personal connection with his
son was still elusive.

"A conflict was that the interruptions really got to me.
Here was this little kid that I truly cared about, yet who
was definitely an interference in my life."

Although his expectations were different, Clarence's
experience was similar. A sensitive, warm-hearted man who
had taken great pleasure in participating in the pregnancy
and birth, he had even arranged for a year's leave from
work in order to be with his daughter full time. He was astonished by his feelings toward her.

"I had a lot of trouble relating to the baby's lack of response and would have to force myself to do things
with her. I was surprised and disappointed at my inability to get right into that. I had expected to be more
emotionally involved from the start."

The common link between the experiences of these
three men was the baby's apparent lack of response. In order to feel comfortable with their babies, these fathers required a kind of behavior they could understand.
Clarence's eyes shone as he remembered when that
finally happened. "All of a sudden they *do* something! Before, they just lie there. The connection came when I began
to see a spark of reaction. It was the baby turning into a
person, something to lock into other than the general joy of
having a child."

Hank described his experience, grinning broadly. "I became aware of the baby responding to me when he would follow me across the room with his eyes. Then I said, 'Right! This is a real person.' It made me feel wonderful. From that moment on the relationship changed."

Actually, babies are highly responsive to human beings from the moment they are born, although their sociability is not immediately apparent. Way before the obvious responses that parents can easily identify, babies are drinking in and reacting to everything they see, hear, smell, touch, and taste. Starting at birth and possibly even before— because it has been established that infants in utero can hear outside sounds—babies respond to human voices. Newborns can see quite well and prefer human faces to other sights. At only six weeks of age, their eyes are sufficiently coordinated to follow moving objects. At eight weeks they can tell their parents apart from strangers simply by looking at them. And by three months, they smile back.

For Seth, those early smiles were the unequivocal expression of connection.

"The first time he smiled at me I figured it was an accident. The next time, I said, 'He *did* mean that look. He *likes* me! He wasn't talking, but he was making jokes and being a person."

The day-by-day development of a baby's sociability is dependent on interaction with human beings. Whenever infants are kissed and caressed, rocked and held close, the touching, motion, and warmth calms them and also helps them to control their body functions. A wonderful spontaneous choreography develops between parents and babies as they respond to and imitate each other with facial expressions, gestures, and sound. Fathers and mothers are equally important in this amazing process, and each, through a unique personal approach, stimulates different areas of social development.

For example, both fathers and mothers talk instinctively to their babies in the special way people reserve for infants—slowly, repetitively, with short phrases. But men tend to react to their babies' vocal sounds by talking back while women are more likely to respond with touching. Men are often more playful with their babies. Women tend to be quieter and emphasize care giving.

Seth noticed how, in response to his playfulness, his son became extra alert and excited.

"Once laughter was part of his repertoire he would screech with glee when we played together. His eyes would get super big, with such intelligence shining there. And his fat little arms and legs would go like the devil with excitement. Every time he learned something new it was an incredible charge."

These male/female variations appear to exist whether or not both parents are involved in baby care. Possibly, as men become more nurturing, their reactions may prove to have been as culturally conditioned as Freud's Victorian responses.

Fathers might be reassured to realize that the first seeds of relating to their babies are sown with early feelings of protectiveness and responsibility, feelings enhanced by the time they spend on infant care. As one man explained, "I learned to appreciate a newborn's helplessness and became more understanding and compassionate."

Built into this tender parental loving is a raw emotional receptivity usually new to first-time fathers, and mothers as well. Over and over men say that they are astonished by the strength of their feelings. These emotions toward their babies are different from anything else they had ever felt. A specific incident may set them off. Such was Simon's experience.

> "The first time the relationship between myself and my daughter hit a substantial level was one day when she fell and hurt her head. The pain for me was overwhelming. I had always loved her before, but it was very undefinable. Now my love became crystal clear."

He went on to observe, "During the pregnancy, I thought only about the joy a baby would bring. Then I realized that the more happiness someone gives you, the more pain you feel also."

Jordan described how his nurturing feelings sharpened. "Walking her all night solidified my feelings as a father. Knowing you're the only one around to provide comfort when she is unhappy or in pain, you start to really care."

From this tremendous vulnerability develops an openness to a deeper connection, a readiness for the special relationship between parent and child, grounded once the baby is seen as a person.

Exclaimed Simon, "I had no way of anticipating how intensely meaningful being with my baby would be. Our relationship has grown into something that enriches me in ways I could never have imagined."

Crying Babies

Babies arrive with personalities, demonstrated in part by their temperaments. Some infants are placid and sleep a lot. Some are alert and calm. Others are restless and cranky. Whatever their disposition, there is just one way for babies to express themselves—by crying!

Most people, when they hear a baby cry, are merely mildly disturbed—but only if that baby belongs to somebody else. A newborn's wails can drive parents up the wall with anguish and irritation.

Eric, the young carpenter, told of the time his son had a stomachache.

"The first time he got sick and was clearly in pain, when he cried I thought he was going to die. We were trying to find out what was wrong. The helplessness of not knowing, the anxiety when what we tried didn't help, waiting for the doctor to call was shattering."

Scott, who had gained in confidence once he became a father, nevertheless spoke of how scared he was whenever his new baby cried.

"Now it's like, if he cries, big deal! But at first it was all 'what if's.' What if he doesn't stop crying, for example. It feels like a life and death situation, though it could be just colic."

Crying is a call for action that sends parents flying to their babies in response. Crying can't be ignored, nor should it be. Attention is crucial to an infant's well-being. Struggling to adjust emotionally and physically to existence outside the womb, helpless to fend for itself, a newborn is totally dependent on others to take notice. Crying is a distress signal that expresses *something*. Response is the cornerstone to the development of a child's security and ability to trust.

In time, crying sorts itself out into decipherable messages: "I'm hungry, tired, sick, uncomfortable, lonely, bored." But until parents have learned to translate, trying to figure out what their baby is asking for can be torture.

Craig shook his head as he remembered his own worry and frustration over being totally in the dark regarding his daughter's needs.

"When you don't know if something is normal or not, there is the anxiety that goes with the soul-searching as you are trying to find answers, the concern over what you are doing, whether you are right or wrong, whether you should be doing something more or less. You internalize everything, externals that don't even relate to the way you are treating the baby."

When Frustration Generates Anger

At times, frustration and helplessness turn to resentment. Compounded by fatigue, resentment can turn to anger. Constantly interrupted sleep is perhaps the toughest sacrifice of all with a young baby, as Hank discovered.

"Working out the nights was the roughest part to live with. He screamed a lot at night. Once I'm asleep, I hate to be wakened. I consider it a direct personal insult. I had to shift a lot of gears to get used to that."

Every parent who has weathered crying and nights of little sleep knows that none of it lasts forever. By the end of an infant's first three months of life even the most devastating behavior is beginning to simmer down. Early on, though, as one father said, "The future is such an unknown, the present so all-consuming, that you see what's happening as going on for a long, long time, which makes it harder to take."

Put together a superabundance of crying and missed sleep with the resentment and frustration they generate, and the predictable result is a pressure cooker of angry feelings. Yet anger at an innocent baby can seem so diametrically opposed to what parents think their emotions should be that they may have difficulty dealing with it. Scott's freelance photography allowed him to work at home part time while his wife went out to work three mornings a week. Sometimes the baby, accustomed to breastfeeding, flatly refused to take the bottled breast milk prepared for him.

"There were times when I was alone with him and he was crying and nothing I could do would make him stop. I just wanted to shake him and throw him out the window. I had to stop myself, put him down, walk out of the room, and let him cry."

Parents who allow themselves to recognize their anger are able to make decisions to avoid reactions that might harm their babies. After several nights of broken sleep, Hank ran out of patience.

"I like quiet. One night, my son slept for two hours, cried for four. The noise, especially in the face of unsuccessful efforts to calm him, made me understand from whence comes child abuse. I definitely felt like it was time to get rid of him. Fortunately, I knew bouncing the kid off the wall wasn't the solution. I felt guilty walking away from him, thinking I should stay with him, but I knew that things were likely to get out of hand. Walking away was safer."

Learning to interpret a small baby's needs takes time and patience. And being able to accept anger as an appropriate response to fatigue and frustration is an essential step toward coping with it. Objectivity helped Eric to appreciate the emotional impact of his anger on his son.

"No matter that my son is still a small baby. He feels my resentment, impatience, tension—everything. So I feel a double responsibility to adjust my controls."

Jordan offered support to his wife, running interference when her anger was running high.

"There is nothing more onerous to me than being dragged out of a deep sleep in a cozy bed. But I noticed my wife's anger, so I'd be up with her."

When parents can confront a situation together, they have a wider range of choices in dealing with it. Non-judgmental discussions with their wives enabled Craig and Seth, whose comments follow, to view their reactions and their situations with an eye toward understanding what was going on and to come up with constructive, even imaginative, solutions.

"There was a safeguard when my wife and I were to-gether because I could give him to her. We took turns getting up and walking outside the house with him so the other one could sleep."

"There were nights when we took him out of the crib and put him between us on the floor, where he couldn't roll off anything. We fell asleep there, while he stayed awake, happy to be near us. With time, we became more relaxed, seeing that kind of thing as an adventure."

For Clarence and his wife, simply riding out the storm was the best alternative.

> "We just weathered the crying and no sleep until it stopped. There wasn't any choice. We kept reminding ourselves that it was a stage that would pass in time. You can't fight it, so you might as well go along with it. I alternated sleeping shifts with my wife and watched a lot of television while rocking the baby. We never got used to it, but we never shut her out either."

Facing anger is harder for a man if he feels that he should be able to be patient and consistent, that it is unmanly to feel inadequate, that he is irresponsible if he takes time out for himself, that other fathers don't feel as he does. For Charlie, it seemed easier at first to ignore the guilt and embarrassment triggered by his resentment toward the son whose presence had changed his life.

> "Looking back from the safety of two years' distance, I realize how frightened I was. I had expected to feel full-time love and tenderness and was horrified by the intensity of my irritability and exasperation. I was so ashamed of that feeling that I couldn't admit it, even to myself."

It is precisely when anger is buried that it strengthens and turns to fury, becoming more likely to explode in actions that can be dangerous. Charlie, who felt shut out and unimportant during his pregnancy, found no change after his son arrived. His wife, who had chosen to breast-feed, was preoccupied with the baby. In addition to the inconvenience of having an infant in the house, Charlie was lonely. He couldn't seem to get acquainted with his son, and his contact with him had dwindled to pinch-hitting for

his wife, especially when the baby—who had a history of
colic—went on one of his crying binges. This is how Charlie
described what happened one spring weekend.

"I had some time off coming up and the forecast was
for sunny, warm weather. We made plans to get outdoors, picnic by the river, stroll through the park. My
wife and I hadn't had a decent outing since my son's
birth eight weeks before, partly because he was such a
fussy baby and demanded so much attention from her.

"Well, this weekend turned out to be no different. He
had whimpered and screamed his way through three
days and two nights. The doctor said it was colic. We
tried all the usual things. It had gotten to the point
where he seemed to be just plain stubborn, refusing to
cooperate just to spite us. By Sunday afternoon I was
exhausted and fed up.

"I was holding him, trying to calm him for the ump-
teenth time when, suddenly, I had had it. Something
blew. I wanted him out of my hands, out of my life. At
that moment I hated him. There was no forethought. I
just threw him, slung him across the room. Some part
of me still in control aimed at the couch, one of those
big, soft cushiony ones, and he landed there unhurt.
My wife was so terrified she couldn't speak.

"I called the pediatrician myself and broke down on the
phone. I felt like I'd broken some kind of non-
negotiable trust, that I'd lost my right to be a father to
this boy, whom I truly did love with all my heart."

Unfortunately, many families go through similar inci-
dents. Charlie had felt emotionally isolated ever since the

pregnancy began. His apparent uselessness during the pregnancy, the distance he couldn't seem to bridge with his wife, his inability to connect with his son, his lack of prestige in his new role—all labeled him a dismal failure in his own eyes. At work, with rough and ready males, where achievement was a primary value and intimacy was limited to, and equated with, sexuality, feelings entered conversations only obliquely. Worst of all, Charlie felt powerless to change anything.

Many new parents, worn down and tired, reach a point where their continuously crying baby, apparently determined not to be comforted, seems to be delivering a direct personal insult. But Charlie couldn't know that. A mutually supportive husband/wife partnership was not available to him, partly because neither he nor his wife knew how to make it happen. Interacting as parents is far different from interacting as lovers.

At times when anger is a problem, it is a prudent and loving decision to call for help *before* the eruption. Pediatricians, visiting nurses, or local health departments are quick sources of information on programs specifically designed to assist parents in handling their anger. Even today, when counseling is common to the point of being fashionable, a man who has been taught to value self-reliance and emotional privacy needs a giant leap of courage in order to admit feeling out of control. Fear of being criticized as unmanly strengthens self-protective barriers. But the shame and guilt of contributing to child abuse is too high a price to pay!

Charlie's heartbroken reaction to what he had done, plus his awareness of what else could have happened broke through his macho armor, and he sought help. "I couldn't believe I was hearing other guys expressing the same things I was going through," he exclaimed. "I felt less like a monster, more like a normal person."

Support groups are not merely for serious problems. All parents need contemporaries with whom to hash over tough times and bad feelings and to share joys, pleasures, and victories. But too rarely does a man have a friend or two with whom he can be completely open about himself without fear of judgment. Fathers' discussion groups can supply this unique companionship.

Fathers speak of various ways to cope with anger. The point to keep in mind is that anger is real and must be recognized rather than repressed. Parents are human beings, not machines. These fathers found that treating themselves with loving consideration helped to make the first months with a new baby happy and healthy for everyone concerned.

"If it got to the point where one of us felt, 'I don't think I can do it any more,' the other came in and saved the day. We used to wonder what would happen if we both decided at once that we couldn't do it. It's a matter not only of tolerating the baby's crying but of caring for your spouse."

"Sometimes when I was up in the middle of the night with my son and feeling overwhelmed, I'd cry. It was allowing myself to feel what I've been protecting myself against. It was responding by moving toward my feelings instead of pulling away from them."

10 Becoming a Family

Talking is a safety valve. Feelings aired are usually less onerous than feelings locked away. Because a man and a woman are sharing the experience of becoming parents, turning to each other for support and understanding seems the obvious thing to do. Ideally, they will explore this new territory together. Clarence knew this:

> "When the friction and tension got to a certain point I just took a deep breath and tried to put things in perspective and cool everything down by talking together."

Realistically, working together may be harder than it seems at first. Throughout pregnancy, the personalities of prospective parents change and shift, readjust, expand. Once the baby arrives, the fabric of a couple's relationship is tested again on a grand scale.

When the family is first at home together, parents shower their full attention freely and joyfully on the new baby.

Eric's experience was a peaceful settling in. "The months before the baby was born, we were so caught up in the expectations, preparations, trying to sort things out, that being with the baby was like a vacation. We had more time to talk to each other."

For Andre, too, in the beginning, "Being wrapped up in the baby was part of the joy of parenthood." After awhile, though, this single focus started to be a strain.

Andre's situation was not an isolated one. For many couples the need to be themselves again edges into the idyllic scenario. Fathers may become aware of problems before mothers do. Andre needed to relate to his wife as an adult, to remind himself that he was still a person in his own right. But his wife remained absorbed in the baby.

> "The first six weeks were easy, like a honeymoon. I was flying high—'I'm a father! This is my son!' I thought I had the world licked. But when the dust settled and I started to get into the old routines, the changes hit. I began to feel that there should be less involvement on her part, that it was time to get back to normal, to resume life as before."

Charlie was glum as he described how severely private time with his wife was rationed.

> "It's tough to get together with your wife because there are so many interruptions. When it was just the two of you, you could sit right down and talk. Now, it might be a week before you get the chance to go on with a conversation you started when the baby cried last Wednesday. And by then I feel, 'Forget it. I don't want to talk about it now. Like, *now* you remember me?' It made me angry that she didn't have time to talk to me right away."

"Normal" to Andre and Charlie, and to many other new fathers who react as they did, means the old one-to-one relationship a man and his wife enjoyed before the baby. But that relationship is gone. Now there are three in the family instead of two.

This is the beginning of parenting—awkward, ignominious, difficult as it sometimes is. For a new father and mother, one aspect of becoming a family is learning to relate to each other within that threesome, as the baby becomes part of their relationship and part of their bond. At the same time, they must make the effort to maintain their identity as a couple. Life with a new baby is akin to undergoing a revolution. The new and the old can blend eventually into a family union, but during the first few months objectivity is hard to come by. The name of the game is adjustment, which takes time, awareness, effort, and patience.

As Kevin pointed out, "The adjustments are continuous, affecting every part of my life except what I do at the office." This picture seems extreme, but as men discuss their experiences the scenario that emerges is anything but unique. It is altogether average.

"It's like being in a giant tug of war," said one father. "On the one hand you are grateful to be blessed with a child, a perfect human being. But on the other, you are grumpy, exhausted, worried, and asking, 'What do I need this for?' "

During those first three months or so, parents can feel trapped by circumstances no longer under their control. There is the baby twenty-four hours a day, a wondrous, demanding stranger capable of causing joy, heartache, and frustrated fury in the space of one minute. A man and a woman, competent adults with well-established lives of their own, see schedules toppled off course, days filled with dirty diapers, smelly burp cloths, unmade beds, cardboard carton meals. Each parent, confused and uncertain, harbors a private suspicion that he, or she, must somehow be responsible for the lack of harmony. It is enough to bring on a case of the blues, and often it does.

New Father Blues

Postpartum blues, as they are known, usually are associated with new mothers and labeled a temporary reaction to the rapidly shifting hormones that conclude pregnancy. But hormones are only part of the picture. New fathers are also susceptible to postpartum blues. Mothers generally experience the blues during the first week after giving birth; fathers may be hit at the same time or not until a few months later.

The blues can take the form of simply feeling low, or they can erupt in full-blown crying jags. They often are particularly devastating because they are usually so unexpected, difficult to identify, and hard to understand. Postpartum depression—often confused with postpartum blues—is a serious, debilitating depression that makes coping with day-to-day living nearly impossible. It is rare. But almost *every* parent experiences postpartum blues.

Sorrow is not an emotion commonly associated with new parenthood. "How could I possibly feel anything bad when everything is so good!" lamented one man. Yet the causes are logical.

Fathers speak of loneliness because they feel distanced from their wives, unconnected with their babies, who add insult to injury by stealing the spotlight. They talk of feeling isolated from their men friends. They mention the unknown, which triggers feelings of inadequacy. Life seems to have gone out of control. And there is no going back. One father points out, "That book is closed." As other fathers explain, sadness is inevitable when certain aspects of life have changed forever.

"The baby has changed my life. It's not that I don't love her. I do, and I am glad she is here. But I mourn the loss of the good old days. Talking about it starts an argument with my wife, so I try being quiet and asking myself, 'Why am I unhappy?' Even to realize that I have to accept that things aren't the way they used to be is scary and shocking. What do you mean, everything isn't hunky dory? It's supposed to be great to have a new baby."

"To come home at night and find her so involved with the baby, it hit me that the days of candlelit dinners for two were over. I suddenly felt such sadness, missing my wife as though she had gone away."

"You start to feel she loves you less. It's frightening. You begin to ask, 'What am I good for? She has the kid; I bring home the pay check.' There's talk and more talk about the child, the child, the child. You get to a certain level, and you'd like to talk about something else. You get a little fed up with the child."

"I'm not number one in the house anymore. We shared in everything. Now that's been taken away. I'm doing lots of things for myself that were done for me before. I had expected to feel lonely until my wife and the baby came home. Instead I feel lonely now they're here."

"I had my spots for things, my way of doing things. My wife had hers. In having a baby I was convinced I was writing off the rest of my life, giving up all my preferences, my freedom to make choices."

The baby's takeover of personal time and space is permanent, not a short-term retrenchment. Each parent, while letting go of a familiar way of life, is also learning to accept the present. This father explained:

> "My feeling was, we'd lost what we had. My question was, would we ever get it back or would we have to build a brand-new relationship? I had to find ways that we were still man and wife."

While there is loss in creating a family, there is also gain. A metamorphosis is taking place. What was originally valuable in a relationship can endure and may improve. Clarence described how the upheaval challenged him to redefine his personal values.

> "Most important, I'm still the same person I used to be. Now it feels like I've sorted through what I used to regard as important, discarded the insignificant, and retained what I truly value. My baby brought me down to earth in a good way."

In working through these changes, it is most important that a father take an active part in current happenings, and that he see his contributions as unique, vital, and constructive. The connections that he develops with his baby, with his wife in their new relationship as parents, and with the new family unit are the very things that can give his new life meaning.

Hank, who had wanted peace and quiet, not parental duties, when he got home from work, was surprised by one of the bonuses built into fatherhood.

"In the past, when my sense of self was getting thinner and thinner, I used to love to go off by myself. Now, if I can't take my son along, I feel cheated."

When Clarence became a fulltime at-home father, he discovered how the soft willingness of the baby to give herself totally to him seemed to convey that, after all, he didn't have to prove himself, that the dreams he felt reflected through her were all possible.

"When times were rough, the baby herself helped. She provided the balance. The baby was kicking off these difficult feelings, but when she did something wonderful, it would make things better immediately."

For every parent involved with baby care, time alone is essential. Fathers, especially those who are at home a lot or who, like Clarence, make arrangements in order to be so, face the same dilemma mothers do—how to get time off for themselves. Seduced by responsibility, concern, and love into marathons of baby care, day after day, parents can become trapped by guilt, seeing time for themselves as an outrageous self-indulgence. But time off provides more than extra sleep and restoring a sense of self. It is a chance to think clearly, to allow free rein to emotions, to reflect on the new life and to assess one's place in it.

"Some of those first fights were over 'Where's that compromise? Where does each of us get our own time slot?' " volunteered Eric, whose decision to become a self-employed carpenter allowed him to share baby care during the early months of his son's infancy. "I found I could cope better with everything if I had that hour on my own."

Work may be the one constant in a new father's changing life. Kevin quite consciously used the time he spent at the office to counteract the strain of life with his new baby. "I need response and acknowledgment to keep myself together," he stated. "When I felt I couldn't handle it any more, work became a place to collect myself. I could leave problems at home."

When men looked back candidly over their early fatherhood, they spoke more of difficulties than of joys. Although they were quick to respond when asked about the pleasure they received from their new babies, adjusting to such an important change in their lives was clearly not easy. This reality needs to be recognized, expressed, and shared for it to be seen as normal. Evolving into a family is often chaotic. Understanding this can help to smooth the way during transition.

Lovemaking with a Baby in the House

When a man feels shut off from his wife because of her closeness with their baby, he may look to lovemaking as a way to bridge the gap. Unfortunately, this form of sharing may be unavailable to new parents. Giving birth interrupts sexual activity only briefly for some couples, but for the majority lovemaking is put aside for several weeks or even months.

Pat explained: "It hit home how very much the physical part of our relationship meant to me. Not sex alone, but all the little things—touching, hugging—that you do as you come into the room or pass each other. Now the baby's needs take away from the energy that would go into 'how are you,' stroking the hair, lying in bed that extra hour in the morning."

Scott said that his wife's disinterest in making love hit him "like a rejection. Her sex drive was almost nil while she was nursing. I particularly missed the intimacy because I saw her so totally involved with the child."

Several factors can affect a new mother's ability to become aroused. Energy is diverted for recovery after the birth and for the conversion of her body to a non-pregnant state. Hormones that contribute to sexual arousal are often diminished or missing, due in part to a temporarily altered hormone balance. Some nursing mothers also find their sexual desire lessened by an abundance of physical and emotional closeness with the baby, and uncomfortably swollen breasts when nursing begins. And most women who have recently given birth experience vaginal tenderness, sometimes for several weeks. As Andre noted:

> "How could she not be tender and sensitive after going through the process of birth? The episiotomy delayed things for a while. If we went slowly and did a lot of cuddling, the soreness let up some, and I could enter her. We had too little leisure for this to happen often."

Fathers may be shocked to discover that they, too, can suffer a loss of libido during the postbirth weeks. Hank couldn't help being affected by his wife's appearance. "I had a problem with the lack of muscle tone," he said apologetically. "She looked like a collapsed party balloon. Her belly felt weird, too, like touching a totally different person. It took some getting used to."

A man's interest in sex can be decreased by fears of hurting his wife so soon after delivery, even when he is assured that this is not the case. Scott explained: "For me, sex had been an unconscious thing, even at its most pleasurable. Now I was more aware and hesitant to act freely in the old ways."

If his wife is nursing, the erratic leaking of breast milk can dampen both bedsheets and ardor. "For me it was a turn-off," said one father. "Not that I cared less about her, but it was a disruption, unattractive to me."

Confronted by new images of themselves as "father" and their wives as "mother," some men have difficulty abandoning themselves sexually. For Simon, sexual awareness and desire seemed unsuitable to his concept of fatherhood. "There was some kind of moralistic issue. When you're a father, you have to be serious, more in control."

Nicholas articulated a response that is familiar to many fathers. Watching his wife give birth transformed his image of her from a sexual partner into that of a powerful female.

"When my daughter first opened her eyes and I saw this consciousness looking back at me, almost indignantly, like, 'Who are you?!' I was awestruck by this opening, the vagina, that had given forth this amazing creature. For several months afterwards, I was a little afraid of dealing with it, this sexual part that I had taken for granted. I was too amazed to get close to it. For two or three weeks after birth I still saw my wife as the great earth mother. Sex didn't feel appropriate, like, 'hands off the sacred vessel.'"

Not all couples lose their sexual desire after their babies are born. For some, as one father put it, there is "no problem. We were eager to begin." But even for these parents there can be restraints. Obstetricians often request that women refrain from sexual intercourse for the first six weeks after birth, the time recommended for the healing of the uterus, vagina, and perineum. Eric recalled, "She was ready much earlier, no leftover soreness at all. But we took the doctor's advice as absolute law. It was very frustrating physically and a hindrance to our being close."

Fatigue is another culprit that curtails orgasm and emotional response, affecting non-nursing mothers and new fathers as well. And, once again, there is concern about becoming pregnant.

Of course, these gloomy reactions are possibilities, not forecasts. In time, parents will get more rest, the whole business of adjusting to parenthood will be easier, and those who have endured celibacy will resume making love. Meanwhile, for many fathers, the absence of physical contact is devastating. Now, as during pregnancy, it is not so much the physical release that they yearn for as it is the emotional connection strengthened through sexual intimacy.

Pat realized the importance of recognizing what lies behind hurt and rejection when overtures to lovemaking are denied. "It can be hard to go beyond being refused to what the act really means," he said. "I miss what making love does for me in terms of bonding or giving me a sense that I'm still valued. It took a lot for me not to get stuck in the hurt, and instead to look beyond it to see the broader issues."

Fathers agree that understanding cause and effect is reassuring. Moreover, when couples make deliberate efforts to stay in touch, they re-establish some of the intimacy they have lost and strengthen their confidence that, eventually, things will settle back to normal. Said these fathers:

> "She was very much less interested in having sex for most of the pregnancy and a long while afterwards. What reassured me the most was that she was as concerned about her loss of libido as I."

> "Due to intense fatigue, lovemaking was clinical for a while, just physical release. I was able to ride with it because I understood it was only temporary. Eventually, the connecting started happening."

As the desire to make love returns, couples are forced to acknowledge that practicality has entered their sex lives. Spontaneous sex has given way to feeding schedules, diaper changes, rocking the cradle. In fact, settling in with a new baby can be so demanding that free time, when it becomes available, is often spent recouping exhausted energy, as Clarence noted.

"On the nights when there was an hour or two after the baby went to bed, my wife would also go to bed. I'd take time for myself, sit down and watch TV. It occurred to me that we could be having sex. But I think we were doing what we each really needed then."

Even the luxury of cuddling and caressing is rare when sleeping babies, apparently endowed with a sixth sense, wake like alarm clocks in the middle of lovemaking.

Seth and his wife felt physically and emotionally ready to resume lovemaking several weeks before anything happened. Something else inhibited them.

"It was as though there was an intruder in the house. The feeling was similar to times when my wife's mother was visiting and sleeping in the next room. For the first four weeks or so we'd say, 'Do you want to start something?', but it never got off the ground."

Even a small baby who sleeps in his parents' room can be given temporary quarters in the living room. But the fact remains that absolute privacy is a thing of the past. Seth remembers:

"Then we realized that it wasn't like when we hold off until her mother goes home. The baby was here to stay. We couldn't wait forever."

Even though the prospect of being interrupted midway through a great love scene by a fussy baby was disturbing, Seth concluded, "It finally occurred to us, so what! The baby will wake up, and the baby will go back to sleep."

With this last obstacle overcome, they were struck by a more basic dilemma. Planning to make love was different from spontaneous sex, unfamiliar and awkward.

"There was a lot of silliness about it, almost like a first date. We were self-conscious."

Being in earnest about their mission, they managed to carry it off and have a lovely time. The baby did wake up, sputtered a few minutes, then dropped off to sleep again. There was a surprising dividend, as Seth and his wife realized over time, something reported by several other parents as well:

"She had become more in touch with her body, freer to enjoy herself. I see the act of birth as a sexual experience. It is totally sensual. I think my wife's freedom is one of the ways it affected her."

The absence of sex during the childbearing year can be an invitation to take sexuality beyond sexual desire to the appreciation of maleness and femaleness as they apply in everyday life. Both parents may experience a new mother's lack of interest in orgasm as a loss of her sense of womanliness. Yet, the womanliness of a woman in the midst of pregnancy, birth, and early mothering is beyond argument. The same is true for a man as he becomes a father. The feeling of being intimately connected as a man and a woman when they make love can be transferred to their experiences as emerging parents.

Nicholas explained how making this important discovery transformed his period of celibacy into an enriching experience.

> "It's like sex when the two of you are very closely in sync, and yet you're still very much in your own gender. In the early weeks I experienced a sense of womanliness in everything my wife did, because it was about being a mother and a woman. And I walked around feeling very intensely male. Under other circumstances abstaining might not be natural, but now it is natural. There's a rhythm to everything. Because there wasn't a release, it intensified the way I felt about everything. I chose to take that intensity and do other things with the baby and my wife. I didn't pretend that I wasn't feeling sexually excited, but I found there was more that could be done with that energy."

There is, of course, no substitute for the private, one-to-one relating that is the heart of every couple's relationship. How to stay in touch is a question that comes up over and over during the early months as parents. As Kevin remarked, "I needed a map to direct me in how to manage time for my wife and me to be together, working around the whims of the baby."

The only solution, say fathers, is to be consciously aware of opportunities to connect, no matter how brief or simple.

"You have to kick in that extra effort, if you want it to work," explained Pat. "Grab your wife, say 'How are you, I love you, hang in there, see you in the morning.' A lot of times I've avoided that because I feel *I* deserve the attention, but you've got to go beyond that."

An evening out is important, too, not merely as two

parents escaping for a few hours, but as two people enjoying each other. Simon laughed. "When we do have time alone—get a baby sitter and go out to dinner and a film— we never get to the film. We wind up talking so, catching up on ourselves."

Andre summed it up: "We shut down sexually for three to four months. It was hard for me. We lost some type of companionship. It's easy to stagnate at home when everything is 'kids.' I found that it was important for us to get together without the baby, even if only for an hour or two, whether it was sex or socializing. You've got to keep doing things together as two people."

The special, personal closeness that a man and a woman enjoy when they have only each other to consider is equally important after a baby comes along. Both the private and parental relationship will be strengthened if they keep sight of this intimacy and strive to achieve it through all the ways available to them, sexual and non-sexual.

11 Pioneering Fathers

Life moves on. Miraculously, the baby is turning into a person, responding with sounds, smiles, and laughter. As a man and a woman become more confident in caring for their child, and their relationship expands to make room for their son or daughter, the trio is on its way to feeling like a family. Craig described how his daughter began to be more an addition than an interruption to their times together.

"During our quiet time, the baby is caught up in the atmosphere. She fits right in, never fusses. When our energy is less concentrated we have to be on the go, paying special attention to her."

For Andre, outings were beginning to be enriched by the presence of his daughter.

"You don't have the time to take off on a Sunday after-noon with a bottle of champagne and lie around for a while, and at the same time it seems less appropriate. Time together is different. There is an intangible change, a good one. We do the things we want to do, and fit the baby in. It never crossed my mind that the baby wouldn't be willing to be a part of things. Maybe that's the reason it works."

The scope of parenting is broadening beyond spelling each other during crying fits or figuring out how to put a tiny arm into a floppy sweater sleeve. Father and mother roles are taking shape.

For many years, these roles were a dependable factor in sorting out which parent did what. Everyone knew that Mother was responsible for child care and housekeeping, appointments with pediatricians and dentists, attendance at nursery school on Parents' Day. Father paid the bills, changed flat tires, shoveled the driveway in winter, and made sure the carpenters shingled the roof properly. If he diapered the baby or kept an eye on him while Mother went to a meeting, he was a nice guy.

These days, rules are loosening up and parental roles are expanding to include all kinds of possibilities. Now Mother can shingle the roof and, although she may receive a wisecrack or two, she is respected for her ability. She can, and often must, bring home a paycheck. She is, in fact, discovering how a career enriches her life. Father, who may turn out to be a better cook than Mother is, isn't laughed at when he appears in the supermarket, baby strapped to his chest, pushing a grocery cart.

Recent focus on self-development and togetherness, plus economic necessity, have joined fathers and mothers in partnerships that are more flexible than ever before. Most exciting, fathers have the option to be as emotionally in-volved and open with their children as they want to be, encouraged by current trends for men to recognize the nur-turing, sensitive, sensual side of themselves.

Andre put into words the sentiments of many fathers today: "Success for me as a man and a father is a lot more than making money. I want an emotionally satisfying rela-tionship with my child from the very beginning, on a daily basis. Being a drop-in father is not for me."

A man is not preordained by society to be a certain kind of father, nor is the way he participates a matter of biology. How he develops his nurturing role is up to him. He will be strongly influenced by his background, his current environment, and, of course, his wife. Ultimately he must define fathering according to the meaning it has for him, not for friends, relatives, society in general, or even his wife.

Take Kevin, for example, who opted for a traditional fathering role. After six months at home his wife returned to her job, teaching high school science. Even though both parents were employed, she was still almost totally responsible for actual baby care.

> "I'll change a diaper once in a while in an emergency, or dress the baby if you show me what to do. But those chores are really my wife's job. I prefer to help out with the marketing and cooking and let her handle the baby care. I'm all thumbs when it comes to that."

Kevin adored his son, loved playing with him, holding him, and taking him for walks. But he drew no satisfaction from the daily routine of daily care and, so, avoided it.

Hank, who felt much the same about baby care, was unable to take such a one-sided arrangement for granted.

> "For a while she did most of the baby care, even though we were both holding down jobs. I had it easy and knew it. Eventually, I started pitching in because I felt it wasn't fair to her."

Hank, like Kevin, had become very attached to his son, spent time with him whenever he could, and was the first to acknowledge that the baby had changed his life.

> "Normally when I get home I take time for myself to relax. But these are the times he wants to play. And it's actually a better way to get rid of what I've been dragging around all day."

Although both of these fathers felt closely involved with their babies, they did not question the division of male and female parenting roles. Even for men who choose to participate equally, new values don't replace old attitudes easily. Lifestyles are relatively easy to rearrange, but traditional concepts of father and mother roles can be so deeply rooted that their existence remains unrecognized.

Simon and his wife had what they regarded as the perfect setup. As a lawyer and an interior designer, respectively, they had been able to rearrange their job schedules to allow each parent long stretches of time with their baby. Yet, as Simon discovered, the influence of time-honored attitudes is subtle and often surprising.

> "We were quite proud of our arrangement, both of us working, baby care fairly divided. When my wife is with clients, I take care of our daughter. And vice versa. What has become an issue is who is to be responsible for the baby when we are both at home. After work, I want to just sit or work alone in the garden. My wife pointed out that I seem to take it for granted that she is primarily in charge of the baby, that I act only as the baby sitter."

Despite their plan, adopted in all sincerity, to share in their daughter's care, Simon saw his role just as Kevin and Hank did theirs—helping out.

In overturning established parenting ideas, the point is not that one parent substitutes for the other, or that everything is done equally or identically. The issue goes beyond who pays the baby sitter or changes a diaper in the middle of the night. Instead, each person's contribution is unique and individual.

According to Scott, it wasn't so much a matter of splitting up chores as it was of respecting each other's capabilities and points of view.

> "I no longer feel like a junior partner of the firm. I used to feel like a hero because I volunteered to take the baby off her hands and maneuvered through the day without her. Now, if I defer to her, it's because she does that particular thing better, not because she's the boss. We consult together instead of apologizing when one of us makes a mistake."

A partnership in parenting has begun. Developing it entails compromise, including a willingness to allow one another room for exploration, and a commitment to stick with trial runs long enough to absorb their flavor. How does each parent feel about taking on the various roles—breadwinner, homemaker, caretaker, nurturing parent—before them? As each partner gains in experience, parenting preferences may shift. The partnership can change as personal interests and needs change.

Clarence and his wife successfully exchanged roles during the first year of their daughter's life. He found getting to know his child first-hand tremendously gratifying.

> "I took a leave of absence and stayed home with her while my wife went to work. I probably had her alone more than my wife did that first year. It was great. I would be very happy not going back to work for another year or two."

In the same way that a husband may be uncomfortable if his wife crosses onto his "turf" by pursuing a career, a woman may resist sharing child care and nurturing, regarding that as her territory. Parenting will then become competitive rather than cooperative.

Studies show that the more a man supports his wife as a new parent, the more capable she is. Logically, the reverse is also true—and is especially important for a father exploring new territory. While he alone determines how he feels, his wife's agreement and support are crucial for him to succeed. The foundation of a parenting partnership must include respect for each other's parenting styles and recognition that each is competent in individual ways.

Craig, who at first observed that extra time spent at home with his wife created tension, now found that "it worked out for the best. We discovered things in each other. She was able to enter my world and understand me better than before from spending so much time together. Our relationship came together solidly, like going from pastel to primary colors."

And Clarence observed that "our respect for each other grew. I learned to be more considerate. I know, before, she wondered 'If this guy has trouble picking up his socks, what's he going to do at two in the morning when the baby cries?'"

Because a nurturing father plays a very different role from the traditional one, his commitment to this approach must be genuine and deep in order to survive and thrive. He may run into conflicts between the personality traits that are useful for career or job and those suited to parenting. A competitive, aggressive, self-focused approach that may be perfect at work is directly opposed to the softly encouraging receptivity and gentle selflessness that characterize time spent with one's child.

In addition, the rewards of a career and those of parenting are vastly different. Job labels often give a man a clearer public identity than does the title of father. Competence may be more specifically appreciated at work than at home, successes more immediately credited. On the flip side, there are jobs that, compared to parenting, may seem dull and unrewarding.

A father who wishes to bridge the gap between work and home worlds may want to change jobs in order to build a life more compatible with nurturing. Whether he takes such a revolutionary step or opts to blend his work and home worlds in other ways, he still faces providing his share of financial support as well as preserving a career that reflects important aspects of himself. He may need to compromise to satisfy both himself and his family.

As a man searches to establish his personal definition of fathering, his present life may contain better examples of nurturing parents—fathers in particular—than his past provides. Any person, male or female, who embodies the qualities a pioneering father values can be a role model. If he must rely only on his own vision, then the clearer it is, the more helpful it will be.

Every man who has been closely involved with his baby directly after birth, if only for a week or so, will have discovered aspects of himself that he can use as guidance. Even Hank and Kevin, whose views were fairly traditional and whose jobs were demanding and time-consuming, found that the foundation had been laid for building a loving, nurturing relationship with their children. Hank highly valued the different person he had become because of his son.

"As a result of having a child, my feeling of detachment has changed, much to my happiness. The process put a large dent in the remoteness that was always a part of me."

Kevin adamantly defined the time he had spent with his baby as father-and-son time. He made it clear that he was *not* filling in for mom. "I don't babysit *my* kid!" he announced. "I babysit *other* people's kids."

For Andre, the bond with his daughter was primary in creating his identity as a father: "It was the developing relationship between me and my daughter that gave me the answers. I stayed open to my feelings as much as I could and tried to let them guide me. You do your best, and whatever happens is the way it should be for you."

Seth, who had been in such a quandary about what it meant to be a father, had this to say when his son was a year old:

> "I believed everything every father told me, including my own. Obviously it was true for them. But after awhile I came to my own conclusions. I had to decide for myself what kind of father to be. I'm still working on it. It becomes clearer all the time."

As men get to know their babies, they get to know themselves. Fathers unanimously testify that having a child changes the way they see themselves and the way they feel about life and the world around them. Hank spoke quietly as he expressed his feelings:

> "I'm more open to show tenderness and to express joy in my son's beauty. I feel more certain of myself as a man, a lot less hung-up about outwardly preserving some kind of machismo image."

Craig, who had been so doubtful about the success of mixing a baby and a musical career, was amazed by what had actually happened.

"Being a father catalyzed me. My feelings of joy affected
my attitude toward work tremendously. In the past I
had enormous fears about my career. I was always
waiting for phone calls. Now I feel like, 'This is me. If
you don't like it, that's cool.' Before, I was more 'Whatever you want, I'll be it.' Being a father strengthened
my sense of self immensely. Financially and artistically
I'm in a lot better position than ever before."

Getting involved gives a father a real chance to fulfill
his potential, not only as a father but as a human being.
Parenting challenges and enriches a man more than any
other role he might tackle in a lifetime. Whether he is drawn
to be a fulltime nurturer, the more traditional provider/
protector/advisor, or a combination of the two, he can still
consider himself a pioneer. Fatherhood is always a venture
into the unknown, a challenge to explore new concepts and
new relationships, an opportunity to expand as a human
being, celebrating the gentler, more sensitive aspects of manhood that stereotyping has overshadowed.

At the end of his first year as a father, Seth summed
up his experience:

"I remember some things so vividly. All the stages, even
the simplest of things, are incredible, flabbergasting.
How quickly they occur and give way to the next! I
look at pictures of him when he was a year, and three
months, and newborn, and I can't remember what he
was like. It seems that he was always as he is now, but
of course he wasn't. It takes all my powers of concen-
tration to bring back the earlier days. Before he was
here I remember very clearly year to year, month to
month. And the birth is like yesterday, every detail,
even what people wore. But the time with the baby is

a blur of wonder and excitement punctuated with hundreds of mental snapshots. Looking back, it happens so fast and is so positive, although at the time you might not see it that way. Everybody warns you about all the terrible times, and we certainly had our share. Overall, to be honest, I didn't expect it to be this good."

Afterword:
A Personal Message

During the two years I worked on this book, I came to feel a strong bond with the men to whom I talked and listened, the many fathers who had conversed with me during my teaching career, and all the unseen, unknown men I now reached out to in my imagination. I realized how my struggles to raise my own son and daughter while developing a career, although highly personal, were neither as unique nor as strictly woman-centered as I had thought. The concerns that hit men so hard when they become fathers were familiar to me, too—having enough money, connecting emotionally with my children, knowing them and myself, passing along values that would enrich and stabilize their lives. I enjoyed relating to the men's assertive, definitive way of thinking, their strength and self-assurance, their ability to laugh at themselves. And I saw vulnerability, sensitivity, passion, and gentleness to match any I'd found in my women friends. Male/female barriers dissolved while, at the same time, my respect, admiration, and delight in these fathers as *men* became clear and powerful.

It seems to me that the clear-thinking, objective, practical, decision-making characteristics of the work world, long equated with masculinity, have their place in the home and can be adapted to situations there, just as the intuitive, supportive warmth associated with a feminine, nurturing home environment has appropriate applications in the work world. I believe that the move by men to be open with their children and, in so doing, to become more fully attuned to their nurturing selves can be the start of an exciting and necessary coming together for families and, even more, for the men, women, and children of the world.

Bibliography

Biller, Henry, Ph.D., *Father Power*, Dennis Meredith, Anchor Press, Garden City, NY, 1975.

*Bing, Elisabeth, and Libby Coleman, *Making Love During Pregnancy*, Bantam, New York, 1977.

*Bittman, Sam, and Sue Rosenberg Zalk, Ph.D., *Expectant Fathers*, Ballantine, New York, 1978.

Bradley, Robert A., M.D., *Husband Coached Childbirth*, Harper & Row, New York, Evanston, London, 1965.

Bruner, Jerome, and Michael Cole, Barbara Lloyd, *Fathers*, Harvard University Press, Cambridge, MA, 1981.

Coleman, Arthur, and Libby Coleman, *Earth Father/Sky Father*, Prentice-Hall, Englewood Cliffs, NJ, 1981.

_____, *Parenting*, Bantam, New York, 1971.

*Eichenbaum, Luise, and Susie Orbach, *What Do Women Want?*, Berkley, New York, 1983.

Garfinkle, Perry, *In a Man's World*, New American Library, New York, 1985.

Grad, Bash, Guyer, Acevedo, Trause, and Reukauf, *The Father Book*, Acropolis, Washington, D.C., 1981.

Green, Bob, *Good Morning, Merry Sunshine*, Atheneum, New York, NY, 1984.

Gresh, Sean, *Becoming a Father*, Butterick, New York, 1980.

Heinowitz, Jack, *Pregnant Fathers*, Prentice-Hall, Englewood Cliffs, NJ, 1982.

McKee, Lorna, and Margaret O'Brien, *The Father Figure*, Tavistock, New York, 1982.

*Panuthos, Claudia, *Transformation through Birth*, Bergin & Garvey, South Hadley, MA, 1984.

Rozdilsky, Mary Lou, and Barbara Banet, *What Now?*, Charles Scribner's Sons, New York, 1974.

Sasmor, Jeanette L., R.N., M.Ed., *What Every Husband Should Know about Having a Baby*, Nelson-Hall, Chicago, 1972.

Schaefer, George, M.D., *The Expectant Father*, Barnes & Noble, New York, 1978.

Steinberg, David, *FatherJournal*, Times Change Press, Albion, CA, 1977.

Stewart, David, Ph.D., *Fathering and Career*, Pennypress, Seattle, WA, 1979.

Sullivan, S. Adams, *The Father's Almanac*, Doubleday, Garden City, NY, 1980.

* Particularly helpful.